NONPRESCRIPTION DRUGS
for the Breastfeeding Mother
2nd Edition

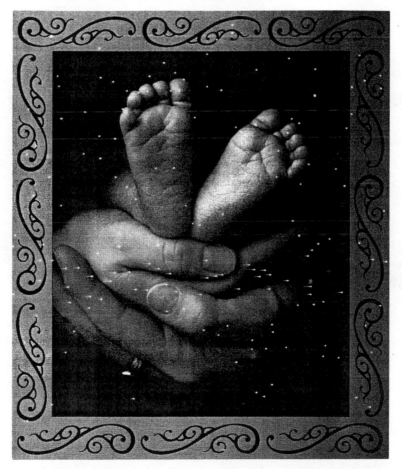

Frank J. Nice RPh, DPA, CPHP

NONPRESCRIPTION DRUGS
for the Breastfeeding Mother

2nd Edition

Frank J. Nice RPh, DPA, CPHP

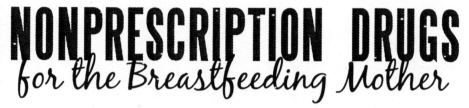

Dear Sarah and Jerre,

Best wishes to you and your family and may God bless you for all you do for Him.

Frank J. Nice

Nonprescription Drugs for the Breastfeeding Mother

2nd Edition

Frank J. Nice RPh, DPA, CPHP

© Copyright 2011

Hale Publishing, L.P.
1712 N. Forest St.
Amarillo, TX 79106-7017
806-376-9900
800-378-1317
www.iBreastfeeding.com
www.halepublishing.com

Cover image: Jessica Crawford

Library of Congress Control Number: 2011920584
ISBN-13: 978-0-9845039-8-8

Printing and Binding: Malloy, Inc.
Cover Printing: Malloy, Inc.

Table of Contents

Dedication vii

Preface ix

Acknowledgement xv

Nonprescription Drugs

Over-the-Counter (OTC) Information Capsules 1

OTC Active Ingredient Categories 7

Nonprescription OTC Drug Labeling 15

Social Drug Overview 17

Nonprescription Drug Tables

Acne Products 19

Analgesic Balms 21

Analgesics, Antipyretics, and Headache and Migraine Products 23

Antacid, Heartburn, Antiflatulant, Digestive Aid, and Activated
Charcoal Products 27

Antidiarrheal Preparations 31

Artificial Sweeteners 32

Asthma Preparations 33

Callus, Corn, and Wart Products 34

Cold, Flu, and Allergy Products 35

Cough and Cold Inhalers, Lozenges, Rubs, and Sprays 46

Dandruff, Psoriasis, and Seborrhea Treatments 48

Heart Attack and Stroke Risk Reduction Agents 51

Hemorrhoidal Preparations 52

Insulin Preparations 54

Laxatives and Stool Softeners 55

Nasal Preparations 58

Nausea, Vomiting, and Motion Sickness Products 61

Ophthalmics (Eye Medicines) 62

Oral Hygiene Products 67

Otics (Ear Medications) 70

Pediculosis (Lice) Treatments 71

Pinworm Treatments 72

Skin Lubricants and Moisturizers 73

Sleep Aid Preparations 79

Smoking Cessation Aids 81

Stimulants 82

Sunscreen Agents 84

Topical Anti-Inflammatory and Anti-Itch Products 86

Topical Antifungals 89

Topical Wound and Burn Care Products 91

Vaginal Products 93

Vitamins and Minerals 95

Weight Management Products 96

Herbs and Dietary Supplements

Herbals 99

Herbal Galactogogues 101

Herbals Commonly Used by Women 105

Herbs Contraindicated in Breastfeeding Mothers and Their
Recommended Alternatives 113

Common Dietary Supplements 115

Breastfeeding and Medications Websites 118

Index 123

Author Biography 149

Dedication

To my wife, Myung Hee, who has graciously supported my breastfeeding counseling over the many years, especially during the innumerable hours spent hovering over my laptop to produce my book.

To my Polish grandparents and parents who sacrificed much to allow me to practice as a pharmacist.

To all the numerous lactation consultants and healthcare professionals and friends and students who have encouraged me over the past 40 years.

To all breastfeeding mothers and children, and especially those breastfeeding mothers of Haiti, whom I have been privileged to serve for the past 15 years. Despite all that you endure as the poorest of the poor, you persevere because breast is best.

You have made my professional career as a consultant pharmacist a true blessing.

Preface

The use of nonprescription or over-the-counter (OTC) medications by breastfeeding mothers is even more common than the use of prescription drugs. The sale and use of these products is a multi-billion dollar industry. Because they are available for common and not-so-common maladies, there is an overwhelming and bewildering variety of nonprescription products available to consumers. Thus, there is always the possibility that a breastfed infant could receive these medications through breast milk, just as with prescription drugs.

The use of a nonprescription medication does not require a doctor's prescription. Therefore, the decision to take a nonprescription medication is almost always made by the mother. Of course, family and friends may influence her decision as to choice. Unfortunately, she may not ask her pharmacist or doctor for advice on the use or its safety of the OTC medication during breastfeeding.

Categories of nonprescription medications that are available to nursing mothers include: acne products; activated charcoal products; allergy preparations; analgesic balms; analgesics; antacids; antidiarrheals; antiflatulants; antipyretics; artificial sweeteners; asthma preparations; callus, corn and wart products; canker and cold sore products; cold preparations; cough and cold inhalers, lozenges, rubs, and sprays; ear and eye medications; dandruff, psoriasis, and seborrhea treatments; dietary supplements; digestive aids; eye and ear medications; flu preparations; headache and migraine products; heart attack and stroke risk reduction agents; heartburn products; hemorrhoidal preparations; herbals, including galactogogues; insulin; laxatives and stool softeners; lice treatments; motion sickness preparations; nasal preparations; nausea and vomiting preparations; oral hygiene products; pinworm treatments; skin lubricants and moisturizers; sleep aid preparations; smoking cessation aids; stimulants; sunscreen agents; topical antifungals; topical anti-inflammatory and anti-itch products; topical wound and burn care products; vaginal products; vitamins and minerals, and weight management products.

In many cases, nonprescription medications consist of multiple ingredients for various symptoms. Many have both regular-strength and extra-strength formulations of the same product. The medication may be short-acting or long-acting. In addition, some mothers may find it difficult to follow complex package directions. They may take an inappropriate medication or may have been given incorrect advice by family or friends. Thus, taking a nonprescription medication may not be as simple as it initially appears. It is certainly more complex for mothers who are breastfeeding.

To assist the breastfeeding mother in determining which nonprescription medications are safe to use while breastfeeding, the following counseling guidelines are offered:

- Avoid taking nonprescription medications for which little breastfeeding information is available. Your pharmacist should be able to assist you with additional information.

- Always choose the safest product to use while breastfeeding. Once again, your pharmacist can help you determine this.

- Take products with single ingredients, rather than multiple ingredient products. It is best for the mother to take a preparation that has one or two specific ingredients that will treat her specific condition, rather than have the mother and her infant be exposed to unnecessary ingredients.

- Use normal strength products rather than the extra strength forms of nonprescription medications. There is no need for the infant to be exposed to extra amounts of a drug when it is not necessary.

- Take short-acting products rather than long-acting nonprescription medications. This protects the infant from being exposed to a drug for a longer period of time, especially if an adverse reaction is possible.

- Know the possible side effects that might occur in the infant, as well as the mother. Your pharmacist can help you with this.

- If possible, as with prescription drugs, the mother should use a nondrug approach to treat her symptoms.

Unfortunately, it is not always clear if it is safe to use a specific nonprescription medication. To assist with decision-making, a series of tables follow. The set of tables was developed based upon those nonprescription products listed in the Physicians' Desk Reference (PDR) for Nonprescription Drugs, Dietary Supplements, and Herbs (2010). Additional commonly used nonprescription medications have been added to these tables. There are literally thousands upon thousands of nonprescription products available for use. It is not possible to list every available preparation. In this work, over 1,700 nonprescription preparations and herbals have been chosen to best represent those that the breastfeeding mother might wish to use. From this list, a breastfeeding mother will be able to select a suitable product that will allow her to continue breastfeeding safely and treat her symptoms.

In most cases, ingredients in ear, eye, oral hygiene, topical (skin), and vaginal preparations do not normally transfer into breast milk in harmful quantities. Topical skin preparations applied to sore or cracked nipples should be specifically indicated for this purpose. Even small amounts of medications applied to the nipple can transfer to the infant, so caution is recommended. Generally, if you can see the medication on the nipple, too much has been used.

Vitamins and minerals in low to moderate doses are generally safe for the breastfeeding mother to take. Pediatric (children's) nonprescription preparations are not in the tables as most mothers would not be taking pediatric medications to treat themselves.

The nonprescription medications presented in the tables represent only the more commonly used products and product categories designated as nonprescription or OTC in the United States. Most nonprescription medications in the United States are also nonprescription in many other countries. Yet, there are some that remain prescription drugs in some foreign countries. Also, product names, dosage strengths, and forms may vary from country to country. Thus, the tables are not meant to be all inclusive or comprehensive for foreign countries.

The following tables provide qualified "Y" = "Yes" and "N" = "No" answers regarding specific nonprescription preparations. The following codes apply to all tables in this booklet:

Y - Usually safe to take when breastfeeding (note any additional cautions)

N - Avoid if at all possible when breastfeeding (note any additional comments)

In addition, Dr. Hale's Lactation risk categories, which are so familiar to the breastfeeding community, have been used with permission.

Dr. Hale's Lactation Risk Categories:

L1 SAFEST:

Drug which has been taken by a large number of breastfeeding mothers without any observed increase in adverse effects in the infant. Controlled studies in breastfeeding women fail to demonstrate a risk to the infant and the possibility of harm to the breastfeeding infant is remote; or the product is not orally bioavailable in an infant.

L2 SAFER:

Drug which has been studied in a limited number of breastfeeding women without an increase in adverse effects in the infant. And/or, the evidence of a demonstrated risk which is likely to follow use of this medication in a breastfeeding woman is remote.

L3 MODERATELY SAFE:

There are no controlled studies in breastfeeding women, however, the risk of untoward effects to a breastfed infant is possible; or, controlled studies show only minimal non-threatening adverse effects. Drugs should be given only if the potential benefit justifies the potential risk to the infant. *(New medications that have absolutely no published data are automatically categorized in this category, regardless of how safe they may be.)*

L4 POSSIBLY HAZARDOUS:

There is positive evidence of risk to a breastfed infant or to Breast milk production, but the benefits from use in breastfeeding mothers may be acceptable despite the risk to the infant (e.g., if the drug is needed in a life-threatening situation or for a serious disease for which safer drugs cannot be used or are ineffective.)

L5 CONTRAINDICATED:

Studies in breastfeeding mothers have demonstrated that there is significant and documented risk to the infant based on human experience, or it is a medication that has a high risk of causing significant damage to an infant. The risk of using the drug in breastfeeding women clearly outweighs any possible benefit from breastfeeding. The drug is contraindicated in women who are breastfeeding an infant.

In this Second Edition, all tables have been updated, expanded, and/ or revised, mainly to include new products, to eliminate discontinued products, and to reflect products that have been renamed. In the current tables, products with the same active ingredients have been listed together, along with the dosage forms for each specific brand name. Information on specific herbals commonly used by women, overall information on herbals, and the list of contraindicated herbals have been expanded and updated. Latin nomenclature has been added for all herbs to better identify specific herbs. Caffeine content of popular beverages has been included in the Stimulants Table. New sections that have been added include a summary of the major OTC categories, a listing of categories of active OTC ingredients, a section on OTC labeling, a Common Dietary Supplements overview, a brief overview of social drugs, and a listing of breastfeeding and medications websites.

Finally, it is important that the mother's healthcare practitioner, in conjunction with the mother, evaluate all the possible risks to the mother and infant. Discontinuing breastfeeding merely to take a medication is simply no longer needed and is not acceptable in most instances. In reality, there are very few drugs that are definitely contraindicated in breastfeeding mothers. The tables in this book were carefully reviewed by experienced clinicians in this field and represent the best data currently available on these nonprescription medications.

THE AUTHOR DOES NOT WARRANT THE SAFETY OF THESE MEDICATIONS DURING BREASTFEEDNIG, BUT ONLY REVIEWS THE CURRENT STATE OF KNOWLEDGE IN THIS FIELD. ULTIMATELY, THE USE OF THESE MEDICATIONS MUST BE REVIEWED BY THE CLINICIAN IN THE FIELD TOGETHER WITH THE MOTHER TO EVALUATE THE RELATIVE SAFETY OF USING THESE PRODUCTS IN BREASTFEEDING MOTHERS.

Frank J. Nice

Acknowledgement

I especially acknowledge my father, Frank Sr., who drove a coal truck, and my grandfathers, Philip and George, who worked deep down in the hard coal mines of Northeastern Pennsylvania. My mother, Irene, and my grandmothers, Sophia and Catherine, all stood by their men as they worked their dangerous trades. Their Polish perseverance ensured that I was the first in my family, not only to attend college, but also to practice as a pharmacist.

There have been numerous lactation consultants, professional colleagues, and students in my life who have encouraged me to continue to help and counsel breastfeeding mothers. They are mentioned in the first edition of the book. Vergie Hughes continues to be my major connection to all matters of breastfeeding. I wish to add Amy Luo from Rutgers University to the list of students who have taught me so much. I thank my fellow pharmacists, Tom Hale, Phil Anderson, and Gerald Briggs, for all the expertise they have contributed to the field of medications and breastfeeding.

My professional career over the years has been outstanding. I thank all my fellow officers who have served with me during my 30 year career in the U.S. Public Health Service and all those who taught me at the Temple University School of Pharmacy, the University of Arizona School of Pharmacy, and the University of Southern California School of Public Administration.

Over-the-Counter (OTC)
Information Capsules

Analgesics, Antipyretics, Headache and Migraine Products

- Analgesics are probably the most common class of OTCs taken by breastfeeding mothers.

- Aspirin has a tendency to cause adverse effects in the infant, especially if used at higher doses. Also, due to the possible link of salicylates with Reye's syndrome, the use of aspirin and other salicylates is not recommended. Low dose aspirin is usually compatible with breastfeeding.

- Ibuprofen is the Non-Steroidal Anti-Inflammatory Drug (NSAID) of choice and has the best safety profile among the NSAIDs. Possessing similar safety profiles, ketoprofen and naproxen are considered usually safe NSAID alternatives during breastfeeding. Do not exceed recommended NSAID doses.

- Acetaminophen is also an analgesic of choice in breastfeeding mothers, since the amount of drug found in milk is relatively small. Do not exceed recommended doses.

Cold, Cough, Flu, and Allergy Preparations

- Overall, antihistamines are reasonably safe to use while breastfeeding.

- Antihistamines may cause irritability or drowsiness in infants. To avoid these side effects, it is best to take antihistamines at bedtime after feeding infants. Also, avoid long-acting, combination, or high-dose antihistamines to help lessen these side effects.

- Decongestants in most cold medications include pseudoephedrine or phenylephrine. Small amounts of pseudoephedrine are found in breast milk, and insignificant amounts of phenylephrine have been reported.

- Mothers taking decongestants may experience a decrease in breast milk production, especially after six months post partum, and should drink extra fluids.

- Guaifenesin (expectorant to loosen phlegm) and dextromethorphan (antitussive to suppress cough) at recommended doses have had no reported adverse events in breastfed infants.

- Alcohol, used in some cough and cold elixirs, can be secreted into milk in concentrations similar to those in the blood. Nursing mothers should avoid any products containing greater than a 20% alcohol concentration to prevent adverse effects.

- Products used for sore throats may contain a variety of soothing agents (camphor, menthol, phenol), local anesthetics (dyclonine, benzocaine), and antiseptics (allantoin). The majority of these products are safe for use, since they are found minimally in breast milk.

- Phenol should be avoided, since safer alternatives are available.

- While naphazoline, oxymetazoline, and xylometazoline are very effective decongestants, they are also long-acting. These products should not be used for more than three to four days in a row. The mother should monitor her milk supply also.

- Phenylephrine is not as long-acting as other nasal decongestants. It is usually safe in breastfeeding; however, the mother should monitor her milk supply.

- No adverse effects have been reported for cromolyn sodium, and it is regarded as a good alternative nasal spray.

- The use of sodium chloride nasal preparations is considered safe.

Asthma Preparations

- It is recommended that asthma products be used only on the advice of a physician.

- Mothers should avoid consuming chocolate, tea, coffee, or cola if using theophylline products in order to prevent excessive stimulation of the infant (e.g., restlessness, insomnia).

Gastrointestinal Agents

- Most laxatives are generally considered safe in breastfeeding, and bulk-forming laxatives (psyllium, methylcellulose, etc.) can be considered first line agents for constipation. These agents are not absorbed from the gastrointestinal tract (GIT), and as a result, do not enter the infant's circulation.

- Senna containing products should be used only for several days.

- No adverse effects have been reported with docusate, a stool softening agent.

- Glycerin suppositories, magnesium citrate, and sodium biphosphate-phosphate enemas are also safe for use.

- Small amounts of loperamide may be found in the breast milk but appear to have no effect on infants. The use of loperamide should not exceed two days for the treatment of diarrhea.

- Attapulgite is safe since it is not absorbed from the GIT.

- The use of bismuth subsalicylate has been investigated in infants and young children with watery diarrhea. The results have led to the conclusion that the amount found in the breast milk should be compatible with nursing. However, because of the unknown risk associated with salicylates and the development of Reye's syndrome, the use of bismuth subsalicylate is questionable and not recommended.

- Antacids are considered safe because the child is exposed to only small amounts of calcium, aluminum, magnesium, and/or sodium from breast milk. They are unlikely to increase bodily concentrations of these minerals, and therefore toxic reactions are unlikely to occur.

- Antiflatulents (for treatment of excessive gas) containing simethicone and lactase are also considered safe for use.

- Simethicone is not absorbed readily by the GIT, and it is also used in colicky infants.

- Lactase is a supplemental enzyme used for lactose intolerance.

- In general, all of the H_2-antagonists are considered safe for use.

- Famotidine and nizatidine are found in lower concentrations in breast milk than cimetidine and ranitidine. Therefore, famotidine and nizatidine are the preferred H_2-antagonists to be used by nursing mothers.

- Any omeprazole ingested through breast milk should be destroyed in the infant's GIT.

Nausea and Vomiting Motion Sickness Products

- The use of antihistamines such as diphenhydramine and dimenhydrinate is usually safe for use in lactating mothers. Infants should be monitored for irritability and/or drowsiness with the use of these antihistamines.

- Limited information on the use of the antihistamines cyclizine and meclizine in nursing mothers is available. As long as other alternatives are available, it would be best, if possible, to avoid cyclizine and meclizine.

- Cola and phosphorated carbohydrates preparations are excellent choices to treat nausea and vomiting in breastfeeding mothers.

- For reasons previously mentioned, bismuth subsalicylate should be avoided.

Hemorrhoidal Preparations

- Hemorrhoidal preparations are used for their local effect; therefore, their use should not result in large amounts of medication in breast milk.

- Preparations include hydrocortisone, cocoa butter, various oils, glycerin, and other ingredients.

Sleep Aid Preparations

- Most of the currently available products contain diphenhydramine. The use of diphenhydramine has been shown to be usually safe and compatible with breastfeeding. Mothers should continue to monitor infants for drowsiness and/or irritability.

- Doxylamine, another antihistamine, is not generally considered to be safe in lactating women, and its use should be avoided and is not recommended.

- For melatonin, a total daily dose of 1 mg to 3 mg appears to be acceptable, although melatonin may potentially interfere with milk production.

Stimulants

- The use of caffeine by nursing mothers is somewhat controversial. Some sources claim that up to two cups of coffee per day will have no effect on the infant, which sounds reasonable.
- Less than 1% of the caffeine ingested by the mother is usually found in breast milk. However, this is not to say that mothers may take large amounts of caffeine without caution, especially with newborns. Increased intake can lead to increased wakefulness and irritability in infants, potentially leading to loss of sleep.

Weight Management Products

- The use of weight management products in nursing mothers is controversial. An important point to remember is that diet and exercise provide a safe and effective alternative to drug therapy. This should be the preferred method for postpartum mothers to lose weight. Since it took nine months to gain weight during the pregnancy, mothers should allow at least nine months to lose weight by using drug free methods such as diet, exercise, and calorie burn-off from breastfeeding.

Artificial Sweeteners

- Aspartame is a commonly used sugar substitute found in many foods, beverages, and OTC products. Milk concentrations of aspartame (and phenylalanine, a metabolite of aspartame) are generally undetectable. Therefore, the use of aspartame in lactating women is compatible with breastfeeding. However, caution should be used with these products in mothers or infants with diagnosed phenylketonuria.

- Acesulfame potassium, saccharin, stevia extract, and sucralose also are safe to take while breastfeeding.

Insulin Preparations

- The use of insulin is common in pregnant women. There are women who suffer from gestational diabetes or diabetes mellitus. After the birth of the infant, the need for insulin may still remain, especially in women with diabetes mellitus. As the result, breastfeeding dose modifications are usually necessary.

- Under the guidance of a physician, the dose of insulin should be reduced by approximately 25% of the prepregnancy dose in order to prevent hypoglycemic reactions in the breastfeeding mother. It is recommended that mothers moderately increase their carbohydrate intake as well.

- There should be no effects of insulin on the infant considering that insulin is degraded in the gastrointestinal tract and does not readily pass into breast milk.

Miscellaneous

- Aspirin is usually recommended for myocardial infarction (heart attack) and stroke risk prevention at a dose of 81 mg or 162 mg. Due to the chemical properties of aspirin at these low doses, the potential risk for Reye's syndrome developing in the breastfed infant should be nonexistent.

- Oral hygiene products are considered compatible with breastfeeding. These products are broken down in the mother's mouth to inert ingredients and are not absorbed into the mother's plasma to any high degree.

- Pinworm treatment medications are not absorbed readily from mothers' gastrointestinal tracts, and thus, only very small amounts of these drugs would appear in breast milk. They are considered compatible with breastfeeding.

- Nicotine replacement products, used as aids to help mothers stop smoking, are usually compatible with breastfeeding. Negligible amounts of nicotine from smoking aids appear in breast milk. The amount of nicotine from the aids is much less than from smoking cigarettes. In addition, none of the other toxic ingredients of cigarettes are present in the aids. Mothers should follow directions explicitly and not smoke when using these products.

- OTC vaginal products used for Candidiasis and yeast infections are usually compatible with breastfeeding. No adverse effects have been shown in babies whose mothers have breastfed while using these medications.

- In most cases, ingredients in ear, eye, and topical (skin) preparations do not normally transfer into breast milk in harmful quantities. Topical skin preparations applied to sore or cracked nipples should be specifically indicated for this purpose. Even small amounts of medications applied to the nipple can transfer orally to the infant, so caution is recommended. Generally, if you can see the medication on the nipple, too much has been used on the nipple.

OTC Active Ingredient Categories

Analgesics, Anti-Inflammatories, and Antipyretics (Oral)
Acetaminophen
Aspirin
Caffeine
Ibuprofen
Ketoprofen
Magnesium salicylate
Naproxen
Phenazopyridine
Potassium nitrate
Salicylamide

Analgesics, Anesthetics, and Anti-Inflammatories (Topical)
Arnica
Benzethonium chloride
Benzocaine
Cajuput oil
Calamine
Camphor
Camphorated phenol
Capsaicin
Clove oil
Dibucaine
Dyclonine
Eucalyptol
Eucalyptus
Hydrocortisone
Ibuprofen
Lidocaine
Menthol
Methylsalicylate
Phenazone
Phenol
Potassium nitrate
Pramoxine
Spearmint oil
Thymol

Trolamine salicylate
Wintergreen oil
Zinc acetate

Antacids and Gastric Acid Reducers

Aluminum carbonate
Aluminum hydroxide
Aluminum trihydroxide
Bismuth subsalicylate
Calcium
Calcium carbonate
Cimetidine
Cola syrup
Famotidine
Magaldrate
Magnesium carbonate
Magnesium hydroxide
Magnesium oxide
Magnesium trihydroxide
Nizatidine
Omeprazole
Phosphorated carbohydrates
Potassium bicarbonate
Ranitidine
Sodium bicarbonate

Antidiarrheals

Attapulgite
Bismuth subsalicylate
Calcium polycarbophil
Loperamide
Pectin

Antiflatulants

Lactase
Lactobacillus acidophilus
Simethicone

Antihistamines

Cetirizine
Chlorpheniramine
Clemastine
Cromolyn sodium
Cyclizine
Diphenhydramine
Doxylamine
Ketotifen
Loratadine
Meclizine
Pheniramine
Phenyltoloxamine
Pramoxine
Pyrilamine

Anti-Infectives, Antiseptics, and Astringents (Topical)

Acetic acid
Alcohol
Allantoin
Allium
Allium aloe
Aluminum sulfate
Bacitracin
Bacitracin zinc
Baking soda
Benzalkonium
Benzethonium
Benzoic acid
Benzoyl peroxide
Benzyl alcohol
Boric acid
Butenafine
Calcium acetate
Carbamide peroxide
Ceresin
Cetylpyridinium
Chlorhexidine gluconate
Chloroxylenol
Citric acid
Citroxain
Clotrimazole

Coal tar
Dimethyl ether-propane
Docosanol
8-hydroxyquinolone
Emu oil
Gamma-hexachlorocyclohexane
Hexetidine
Hydantoin
Hydrogen peroxide
Ichthammol
Isopropyl alcohol
Ketoconazole
Lindane
Magnesium peroxide
Miconazole
Natrum muriaticum
Natural oil extracts
Neomycin
Octocrylene
Pyrethrum extract
Permethrin
Peroxide
Piperonyl butoxide
Polymyxin B
Polymyxin B sulfate
Povidone iodine
Pyrantel pamoate
Pyrithione zinc
Salicylic acid
Selenium sulfide
Sodium borate
Sodium oxychlorosene
Sodium perborate monohydrate
Sulfur
Terbinafine
Tetrasodium pyrophosphate
Tioconazole
Tolnaftate
Triclosan
Undecylenic acid
Vinegar
Zinc chloride
Zinc sulfate
Zincum oxydatum

Antitussives and Expectorants

Dextromethorphan
Guaifenesin
Menthol
Potassium guaiacolsulfonate
Potassium iodide

Artificial Sweeteners

Acesulfame potassium
Aspartame
Saccharin
Sodium saccharin
Stevia extract
Sucralose

Decongestants

Antazoline
Levmetamfetamine
Naphazoline
Oxymetazoline
Phenylephrine
Propylhexedrine
Pseudoephedrine
Tetrahydrozoline
Xylometazoline

Diuretics

Pamabrom

Laxatives and Stool Softeners

Bisacodyl
Calcium polycarbophil
Cascara sagrada
Castor oil
Dibasic sodium phosphate
Docusate calcium
Docusate sodium
Glycerin
Magnesium citrate

Magnesium hydroxide
Methylcellulose
Mineral oil
Monobasic sodium phosphate
Picosulphate
Potassium bitartrate
Potassium sorbate
Psyllium
Rhubarb
Saline
Senna
Sennosides
Sodium propionate

Lubricants, Moisturizers and Protectants

Aloe
Aminobenzoic acid
Ammonium lactate
Avobenzone
Bentoquatam
Benzophenone-9
Caprylic-capric triglyceride
Carboxymethylcellulose
Chamomile
Cinoxate
Cocoa butter
Cod liver oil
Colloidal oatmeal
Compound benzoin tincture
Corn starch
Dextran
Dimethicone
Dioxybenzone
Ecamsule
Giant kelp leaf extract
Glycerin
Glycerol
Homosalate
Hydroxypropyl methylcellulose
Hypromellose
Isopenyl-4-methoxycinnamate
Lactic acid
Lanolin

Lanolin oil
Methyl anthranilate
Methylbenzylidene camphor
Mexoryl XL
Mineral oil
Neo Heliopan AP
Oat kernel extract
Oatmeal
Octocrylene
Octyl methoxycinnamate
Octyl salicylate
Oxybenzone
PABA
Padimate O
Parsol SLX
PEG-6-32
PEG-20
PEG-40
Peruvian balsam
Petrolatum
Phenylbenzimidazole sulfonic acid
Polycarbophil
Polyethylene glycol 400
Polysorbate 80
Polyvinyl alcohol
Potassium lactate
Povidone
Propylene glycol
Shark liver oil
Shea butter
Sodium chloride
Sodium hyaluronate
Sodium lactate
Sulisobenzone
Sunflower oil
Tinosorb M
Tinosorb S
Titanium oxide
Topical starch
Trolamine salicylate
Urea
Uvasorb HEB
Uvinul A Plus
Uvinul T 150

Vitamin A
Vitamin D
Vitamin E
White petrolatum
Witch hazel
Zinc oxide

Nonprescription OTC Drug Labeling

It is very important to read the label when using nonprescription OTC drugs. Labeling helps ensure that drugs are used correctly and safely. The FDA has issued new regulations regarding OTC drug labeling. The regulations will enable consumers to choose the best and safest way to use OTC drugs. Consumers using the labeling information, in addition to information provided in this book, will maximize the safety and compatibility of selected nonprescription products during breastfeeding.

How is the new labeling different?

- The label uses common words that are easy to understand.
- The print is larger, making it easier to read.
- The label looks the same for all products and is in the same place, on every product.

How does the label help the consumer?

- The label helps the consumer compare products and choose the best one for the consumer's specific illness or condition.
- The product will work its best because the consumer can use it correctly based on the labeling information.
- The consumer will have all the necessary information needed to avoid potential problems.

What is on the label?

- **Active ingredient.** The active ingredient is the chemical compound in the medicine that works to relieve your symptoms. It is always the first item on the label. There may be more than one active ingredient in a product. The label will clearly show this, and it will also show the purpose of each active ingredient. It is usually best for breastfeeding mothers to take single active ingredient products. To reduce your risk and your baby's risk of overdose, be sure to check that you're not taking two medicines that contain the same ingredients or are intended for the same purpose.

Note: Active ingredients for each nonprescription drug product are listed in the tables in this book.

- **Uses.** This section lists the symptoms the medicine is meant to treat. Uses are sometimes called "indications."

- **Warnings.** This safety information will tell you what other medicines, foods, or activities (such as driving) to avoid while taking this medicine, as well as possible side effects of taking the medicine. The warning will also tell you if the medicine is not recommended for a particular group of people, such as pregnant women.

- **Directions.** This section tells you how much medicine you should take, how often you should take it, and for how long you can take it. The directions may be different for children and adults.

- **Other information.** Any other important information, such as how to store the medicine, will be listed here.

- **Inactive ingredients.** An inactive ingredient is a chemical compound in the medicine that isn't meant to treat a symptom. This can include preservatives, binding agents, and food coloring. This section is especially important for people who know they or their babies have allergies to food coloring or other chemicals.

Note: Inactive ingredients are not listed for each nonprescription drug product in the tables in this book; carefully read all ingredients listed on the label.

- **Questions or Comments.** A toll-free number for the manufacturer is provided in case you have any questions or want to share your comments about the medicine.

Social Drug Overview

Caffeine

- Even though clearance of caffeine in infants is markedly reduced, caffeine ingested through breast milk by nursing children is usually insignificant, if reasonable amounts (1 cup to 2 cups per day) of coffee, tea, and/or caffeine-containing soft drinks are used by the mother. See Table on page 85 for amounts of caffeine in these drinks.

- Mothers of newborns, and in particular of premature newborns, should avoid caffeine.

- If taking theophylline containing products, mothers should avoid drinks containing caffeine.

Alcohol

- One to two cocktails, glasses of wine, or bottles of beer usually result in insignificant levels of alcohol in breast milk.

- The odor of alcohol in milk may cause infants to consume significantly less milk.

- Excessive, chronic drinking can result in mild sedation to deep sleep and/or hypoprothrombinemic bleeding in infants.

- Intoxicated mothers should not breastfeed; chronic alcoholics should not breastfeed.

Nicotine

- Vomiting, diarrhea, tachycardia, and restlessness were reported in a breastfed infant in a 1937 case study when a mother smoked 20 cigarettes per day.

- Nicotine and toxic byproducts are rapidly transferred into breast milk with a long half-life of approximately 90 minutes.

- Many other contaminants, along with nicotine, are present in cigarettes.

- Cigarettes may have a negative influence on breast milk volume and affect the energy requirements of breastfed infants.

- Nicotine patches are safe to use, but the mother must not smoke on the side.

Acne Products

Aveeno Clear Complexion Bar/Clear Complexion Foaming Cleanser (salicylic acid)	Y	L2
Benzoyl Peroxide Bar/Cleanser/Cream/Gel/Wash (benzoyl peroxide)	Y	L1
Biore Blemish Fighting Ice Cleanser (salicylic acid)	Y	L2
Clean & Clear Advantage Acne Spot Treatment/Advantage Oil-Free Acne Moisturizer/Blackhead Clearing Daily Cleansing Pads/Blackhead Cleansing Scrub/Continuous Control Acne Wash Oil-Free (salicylic acid)	Y	L2
Clean & Clear Continuous Control Acne Cleanser/Persia-Gel 10 Maximum Strength (benzoyl peroxide)	Y	L1
Clearasil Acne Treatment Tinted Cream/Stay Clear Vanishing Acne Treatment Cream/Total Acne Control/Ultra Acne Rapid Action Treatment Vanishing Cream (benzoyl peroxide)	Y	L1
Clearasil Stay Clear Acne Fighting Cleansing Wipes/Stay Clear Daily Facial Scrub/Stay Clear Daily Pore Cleansing Pads/Stay Clear Stay Clear Oil-Free Gel Wash/Stay Clear Skin Perfecting Wash/Ultra Acne Clearing Gel Wash/Ultra Acne Clearing Scrub/Ultra Daily Face Wash/Ultra Deep Pore Cleansing Pads (salicylic acid)	Y	L2
Neutrogena Acne Stress Control 3-in-1 Hydrating Acne Treatment/Advanced Solutions Acne Mark Fading Peel with CelluZyme/Blackhead Eliminating Daily Scrub/Blackhead Eliminating Foaming Pads/Body Clear Body Scrub/Clear Pore Oil-Eliminating Astringent/Oil Free Acne Stress Control Power Clear Scrub/Oil Free Acne Wash Cleansing Cloths/Oil Free Acne Wash Cream Cleanser/Oil Free Acne Wash Foam Cleanser/Oil Free Anti-Acne Moisturizer/Rapid Clear Acne Defense Face Lotion/Triple Clean Anti-Blemish Astringent/Triple Clean Anti-Blemish Pads (salicylic acid)	Y	L2
Neutrogena Clear Pore Cleanser Mask/On-the-Spot Acne Treatment Vanishing Formula (benzoyl peroxide)	Y	L1

Noxzema Triple Clean Anti-Bacterial Lathering Cleanser (triclosan)	Y	L1
Olay Body Wash/Chill Factor Cleansing Pads/Daily Facials Lathering Cleansing Cloths-Clarifying for Combination-Oily Skin/Maximum Daily Cleansing Pads/Maximum Face Scrub/Regenerist Daily Regenerating Cleanser/Total Effects Plus Blemish Control Moisturizer (salicylic acid)	Y	L2
Oxy Chill Factor Daily Wash/Maximum Daily Wash/Spot Treatment (benzoyl peroxide)	Y	L1
PanOxyl Aqua Gel Maximum Strength Gel/Bar 10% Maximum Strength/Facial Bar 5% (benzoyl peroxide)	Y	L1
Phisoderm Anti-Blemish Body Wash (salicylic acid)	Y	L2
St. Ives Medicated Apricot Scrub (salicylic acid)	Y	L2
Stridex Essential Pads with Salicylic Acid/Facewipes to Go with Acne Medication/Maximum Strength Alcohol Free/Sensitive Skin Pads Alcohol Free (salicylic acid)	Y	L2
ZAPZYT Acne Wash Treatment For Face & Body/Pore Treatment Gel (salicylic acid)	Y	L2
ZAPZYT Maximum Strength Acne Treatment Gel/Treatment Bar (benzoyl peroxide)	Y	Li

Y   Usually safe when breastfeeding
L1-L5 Hale's Lactation Risk Category

Analgesic Balms

Absorbine Jr. Back Patch/Back Ultra Strength Patch/Liniment (menthol/thymol)	Y1	L2
ActivOn Ultra Strength Backache Roll-On Liquid (camphor/menthol)	Y1	L2
ArthriCare Cream (capsaicin)	Y1	L3
Arthritis Hot Crème (menthol/methylsalicylate)	Y1	L3
Axsain Cream (capsaicin)	Y1	L3
Aspercreme Cream/Lotion (trolamine salicylate)	Y1	L3
Bengay Arthritis Cream (menthol/methylsalicylate)	Y1	L3
Bengay Cream (camphor/menthol/methylsalicylate)	Y1	L3
Capzasin-HP Crème (capsaicin)	Y1	L3
CM Plex Cream (cetylated fatty acids/fish oil/soy)	Y1	L1
Flexall 454 Gel/454 Maximum Strength Gel (menthol)	Y1	L1
Flexall Plus Maximum Strength Gel (camphor/menthol/methylsalicylate)	Y1	L3
Icy Hot Cream/Patch XL/Roll/Sleeve/Stick (menthol/methylsalicylate)	Y1	L3
Infrarub Ointment (capsaicin)	Y1	L3
JointFlex Cream/Ice Roll-On (camphor)	Y1	L2
Mineral Ice Gel (menthol)	Y1	L2
Myoflex Cream (trolamine salicylate)	Y1	L3
Sportscreme Cream (trolamine salicylate)	Y1	L3
Nuprin Cream (ibuprofen)	Y1	L1
Salonpass Arthritis Pain Patch/Pain Relief Patch (menthol/methylsalicylate)	Y1	L3
Thera-Gesic Cream (menthol/methylsalicylate)	Y1	L3
Tiger Balm (cajuput oil/camphor/clove oil/menthol)	Y1	L2
Topricin Cream (arnica)	Y1	L3
Traumeel Ointment (arnica)	Y1	L3

Trixaicin HP Cream (capsaicin)	Y1	L3
Zostrix Arthritis Cream (capsaicin)	Y1	L3

Y1   Usually safe when breastfeeding (do not apply to breasts)

Analgesics, Antipyretics, and Headache and Migraine Products

Acetaminophen Tablets (acetaminophen)	Y	L1
Actidose with Sorbitol Suspension (activated charcoal/ sorbitol)	Y	L1
Actidose-Aqua Suspension (activated charcoal)	Y	L1
Advil Caplets/Gel Caplets/Liqui-Gels/Migraine Capsules/Tablets (ibuprofen)	Y	L1
Aleve Caplets/Liquid Gels/Smooth Gels/Tablets (naproxen)	Y	L3
Alka-Seltzer Effervescent Antacid and Pain Reliever Original Tablets/Extra Strength Tablets (aspirin/sodium bicarbonate)	N	L4
Alka-Seltzer Morning Relief Tablets/Wake-Up Call Tablets (aspirin/caffeine)	N	L4
Anacin Advanced Headache Tablets (acetaminophen/ aspirin/caffeine)	N	L4
Anacin Fast Pain Relief Tablets/Maximum Strength Tablets/Tablets (aspirin/caffeine)	N	L4
Anacin Aspirin Free Extra Strength Tablets (acetaminophen)	Y	L1
Arthritis Pain Relief Caplets (acetaminophen)	Y	L1
Ascriptin Maximum Strength Tablets/Regular Strength Tablets (aluminum-magnesium hydroxide/ aspirin/ calcium carbonate)	N	L4
Aspercin Tablets (aspirin)	N	L4
Aspirin 325 mg Tablets (aspirin)	N	L4
Aspirin 500 mg Tablets (aspirin)	N	L4
Aspirin Free Pain Relief Tablets (acetaminophen)	Y	L1
Back-Quell Tablets (acetaminophen/magnesium salicylate)	N	L4
Bayer Back & Body Pain Caplets (aspirin/caffeine)	N	L4

Bayer Extra Strength Caplets/Genuine Tablets/Safety Coated Caplets (aspirin)	N	L4
Bayer Extra Strength Plus Caplets (aspirin/calcium carbonate)	N	L4
BC Arthritis Strength Powders/Original Strength Powders (aspirin/caffeine/salicylamide)	N	L4
Bromo-Seltzer Powders (acetaminophen/citric acid/ sodium bicarbonate)	Y2	L1
Bufen Tablets (ibuprofen)	Y	Y1
Bufferin Extra Strength Tablets (aspirin/calcium-magnesium carbonate/magnesium oxide)	N	L4
Bufferin Tablets (aspirin/benzoic-citric acid)	N	L4
Datril Tablets (acetaminophen)	Y	L1
DeWitt's Pills Tablets (magnesium salicylate)	N	L4
Doan's Extra Strength Caplets (magnesium salicylate)	N	L4
Dynafed IB Tablets/Tablets EX (acetaminophen)	Y	L1
Dyspel Tablets (acetaminophen/pamabrom/pyridoxine)	Y2, Y3	L3
Ecotrin Regular Strength Tablets (aspirin)	N	L4
Emagrin Tablets (aspirin/caffeine/salicylamide)	N	L4
Empirin Tablets (aspirin)		
Excedrin Back & Body Capsules (acetaminophen/ aspirin buffered)	N	L4
Excedrin Extra Strength Caplets/Extra Strength Express Gels/Extra Strength Geltabs/Extra Strength Tablets/ Migraine Caplets/Migraine Geltabs/Migraine Tablets (acetaminophen/aspirin)	N	L4
Excedrin Tension Headache Caplets/Tension Headache Express Gels/Tension Headache Geltabs (acetaminophen/caffeine)	Y1, Y2	L2
EZ-Char Pellets (activated charcoal)	Y	L1
Feverall Adult Strength Suppository (acetaminophen)	Y	L1
Goody's Body Pain Formula Powders (acetaminophen/ aspirin)	N	L4

24

Goody's Extra Cool Orange Powders/Extra Strength Headache Powders (acetaminophen/aspirin/caffeine)	N	L4
Haltran Tablets (ibuprofen)	Y	L1
Healthprin Full Strength Tablets (aspirin)	N	L4
Hyland's Leg Cramps with Quinine Caplets/Sublingual Tablets (herbs/magnesium/quinine)	N	L4
Hyland's Restful Legs Tablets (herbs)	N	L4
Ibuprofen 200 mg Tablets (ibuprofen)	Y	L1
Ibuprohm Max Tablets/Tablets (ibuprofen)	Y	L1
Ibuprom Max Tablets (ibuprofen)	Y	L1
Magsal Tablets (magnesium salicylate/ phenyltoloxamine)	N	L4
Midol Menstrual Complete Caplets/Menstrual Complete Gelcaps (acetaminophen/caffeine/pyrilamine)	Y1, Y2	L3
Midol Teen Formula Caplets (acetaminophen/ pamabrom)	Y2, Y3	L3
Midol IB Cramp Relief Formula Tablets (ibuprofen)	Y	L1
Mobigesic Tablets (magnesium salicylate/ phenyltoloxamine)	N	L4
Motrin IB Caplets/Tablets (ibuprofen)	Y	L1
Nuprin Tablets (ibuprofen)	Y	L1
Orudis KT Capsules (ketoprofen)	Y	L3
Pamprin All Day Caplets (naproxen)	Y	L3
Pamprin Cramp Caplets (acetaminophen/magnesium salicylate/pamabrom)	N	L4
Pamprin Max Caplets (acetaminophen/aspirin/caffeine)	N	L4
Pamprin Multi-Symptom Caplets (acetaminophen/ pamabrom/pyrilamine)	N	L4
Panadol Tablets (acetaminophen)	Y	L1
Panadol Extra Tablets (acetaminophen/caffeine)	Y1, Y2	L2
Percogesic Extra Strength Caplets/Original Strength Caplets (acetaminophen/phenyltoloxamine)	N	L4

Premsyn PMS Caplets (acetaminophen/pamabrom/ pyrilamine)	Y1, Y2, Y3	L3
Prodium Tablets (phenazopyridine)	Y	L3
Re-Azo Tablets (phenazopyridine)	Y	L3
Stanback Headache Powders (aspirin/caffeine/ salicylamide)	N	L4
Supac Tablets (acetaminophen/aspirin/caffeine)	N	L4
Tylenol Arthritis Caplets/Arthritis Geltabs/8 Hour Caplets/Extra Strength Caplets/Extra Strength Cool Caplets/Extra Strength EZ Tablets/Extra Strength Rapid-Release Gelcaps/Extra Strength Rapid Blast Liquid/Regular Strength Tablets (acetaminophen)	Y	L1
Traumeel Oral Drops (herbs)	N	L4
Traumeel Oral Liquid in Vials (herbs)	N	L4
Traumeel Tablets (herbs)	N	L4
Ultraprin Tablets (ibuprofen)	Y	L1
Uristat Tablets (phenazopyridine)	Y	L3
Vanquish Caplets (acetaminophen/aspirin/caffeine)	N	L4

Y *Usually safe when breastfeeding*
Y1 *Usually safe when breastfeeding (monitor infant for drowsiness and/ or excitability)*
Y2 *Usually safe when breastfeeding (best taken as individual ingredients to treat only specific symptoms)*
Y3 *Usually safe when breastfeeding (monitor for decrease milk production; mother should drink extra fluids)*
N *Avoid when breastfeeding*

Antacid, Heartburn, Antiflatulant, Digestive Aid, and Activated Charcoal Products

Alka-Mints Tablets (calcium carbonate)	Y	L1
Alka-Seltzer Extra Strength Tablets/Lemon Lime Tablets/ Original Tablets (aspirin/citric acid/sodium bicarbonate)	N	L4
Alka-Seltzer Gold Tablets (citric acid/potassium-sodium bicarbonate)	Y	L1
Alka-Seltzer Heartburn Relief Tablets (citric acid/sodium bicarbonate)	Y	L1
Alkets Tablets (calcium carbonate)	Y	L1
AlternaGEL Liquid (aluminum hydroxide)	Y	L1
Alu-Cap Capsules (aluminum hydroxide)	Y	L1
Alu-Tab Tablets (aluminum hydroxide)	Y	L1
Aludrox Liquid (aluminum hydroxide)	Y	L1
Amitone Tablets (calcium carbonate)	Y	L1
Amphogel (aluminum hydroxide)	Y	L1
Axid Capsules (nizatidine)	Y	L1
Axid AR Tablets (nizatidine)	Y	L2
Basaljel Liquid (aluminum carbonate)	Y	L1
Beano Food Enzyme Dietary Supplemental Drops/ Food Enzyme Dietary Supplemental Tablets (alpha-galactosidase enzyme)	Y	L1
Beano Meltaways/Tablets (enzymes/sorbitol)	Y	L1
BeSure Prevent Gas Capsules (food enzymes)	Y	L1
Brioschi Powders (sodium bicarbonate/tartaric acid)	Y	L1
Chooz Gum Tablet (calcium carbonate)	Y	L1
Citrocarbonate Effervescent Antacid Salts (sodium bicarbonate-citrate)	Y	L1
Dairy Ease Capsules (lactase)	Y	L1

DairyEnz Capsules (lactase)	Y	L1
DairyGest Lactozymes Capsules (lactase)	Y	L1
DDS-Acidophilus Capsules (lactobacillus acidophilus)	Y	L1
Dicarbosil Tablets (calcium carbonate)	Y	L1
Di-Gel Tablets (calcium carbonate/magnesium hydroxide/ simethicone)	Y	L1
GasAid Maximum Strength Anti-Gas Softgels (simethicone)	Y	L1
Gas-X Antigas Chewable Tablets/Antigas Softgels/Antigas Thin Strips (simethicone)	Y	L1
Gas-X Extra Strength with Maalox Chewable Tablets (calcium carbonate/simethicone)	Y	L1
Gaviscon Regular Strength Liquid/Extra Strength Tablets/Regular Strength Liquid/Regular Strength Tablets (aluminum hydroxide/magnesium carbonate)	Y	L1
Gelusil Chewable Tablets (aluminum-magnesium hydroxide/simethicone)	Y	L1
Lactaid Fast Act Capsules/Fast Act Chewable Tablets/ Original Tablets (lactase enzymes)	Y	L1
Lactase Capsules (lactase)	Y	L1
Lactinex Granules/Tablets (lactobacillus culture)	Y	L1
Liquid Lactase Drops (lactase)	Y	L1
Maalox Advanced Maximum Strength Chewable Tablets (calcium carbonate/simethicone)	Y	L1
Maalox Advanced Maximum Strength Liquid/Advanced Regular Strength Liquid (aluminum-magnesium hydroxide/simethicone)	Y	L1
Maalox Regular Strength Chewable Tablets (calcium carbonate)	Y	L1
Maalox Total Relief Maximum Strength Relief Liquid (bismuth subsalicylate)	N	L4
Mylanta Gas Maximum Strength Chewable Tablets/ Softgels (simethicone)	Y	L1
Mylanta Maximum Strength Liquid/Regular Strength Liquid (aluminum-magnesium hydroxide/simethicone)	Y	L1

Mylanta Supreme Antacid Liquid (aluminum-magnesium hydroxide)	Y	L1
Mylanta Ultimate Strength Chewable Tablets/Ultimate Strength Liquid (calcium carbonate/magnesium hydroxide)	Y	L1
Nephrox Suspension (aluminum hydroxide/mineral oil)	Y	L1
Pepcid AC Gelcaps/Maximum Strength Chews/Maximum Strength Tablets/Tablets (famotidine)	Y	L2
Pepcid Complete Chewable Tablets (calcium carbonate/ famotidine/magnesium carbonate)	Y	Y2
Pepto-Bismol Caplets/Cherry Maximum Strength Liquid/Instacool Peppermint Chewable Tablets/Maximum Strength Liquid/Original Chewable Tablets/Original Liquid (bismuth subsalicylate)	N	L4
Phazyme 95 Capsules/Tablets (simethicone)	Y	L1
Phillips Milk of Magnesia Suspension/Tablets (magnesium hydroxide)	Y	L1
Prilosec OTC Tablets (omeprazole)	Y	L2
Riopan Plus Suspension/Plus Tablets (magaldrate/ simethicone)	Y	L1
Rolaids Antacid & Antigas Soft Chews (calcium carbonate/simethicone)	Y	L1
Rolaids Extra Strength Plus Gas Soft Chews (calcium carbonate/simethicone)	Y	L1
Rolaids Extra Strength Soft Chews (calcium carbonate)	Y	L1
Rolaids Extra Strength Tablets/Tablets (calcium carbonate/ magnesium hydroxide)	Y	L1
Rolaids Multi-Symptom Chewable Tablets (calcium carbonate/magnesium hydroxide/simethicone)	Y	L1
Sodium Bicarbonate Powder/Tablets (sodium bicarbonate)	Y	L1
Tagamet HB Tablets (cimetidine)	Y	L2
Titralac Chewable Tablets (calcium carbonate)	Y	L1
Titralac Plus Chewable Tablets (calcium carbonate/ simethicone)	Y	L1

Tums Chewable Tablets/E-X 750 Chewable Tablets/E-X 750 Sugar Free Chewable Tablets/Smoothies Tablets/Ultra 1000 Chewable Tablets (calcium carbonate)	Y	L1
Zantac 75 Tablets (ranitidine)	Y	L2
Zantac 150 Tablets (ranitidine)	Y	L2
Zegerid OTC Tablets (omeprazole/sodium bicarbonate)	Y	L2

Y   *Usually safe when breastfeeding*
N   *Avoid when breastfeeding*

Antidiarrheal Preparations

Diar Aid Caplets (loperamide)	Y1	L2
Diar Aid Tablets (attapulgite/pectin)	Y	L1
Diarrest Tablets (attapulgite)	Y	L1
Diasorb Capsules (loperamide)	Y1	L2
Diasorb Tablets (attapulgite)	Y	L1
Diatrol Tablets (attapulgite)	Y	L1
Donnagel Suspension (attapulgite)	Y	L1
Equalactin Chewable Tablets (calcium polycarbophil)	Y	L1
Hyland's Diarrex Tablets (herbs)	N	L4
Fibercon Caplets (calcium polycarbophil)	Y	L1
Imodium A -D Caplets/E-Z Chews/Liquid (loperamide)	Y1	L2
Imodium Multi-Symptom Relief Caplets/Multi-Symptom Relief Chewable Tablets (loperamide/simethicone)	Y1	L2
K-Pek Suspension (attapulgite)	Y	L1
Kao-Paverin Capsules (loperamide)	Y1	L2
Kaopek Suspension (attapulgite)	Y	L1
Kaopectate Advanced Formula Suspension/Maximum Strength Tablets/Tablets (attapulgite)	Y	L1
Kaopectate Extra Strength Liquid/Liquid (bismuth subsalicylate)	N	L3
Konsyl Fiber Caplets (calcium polycarbophil)	Y	L1
Maalox Total Relief Liquid (bismuth subsalicylate)	N	L3
Parepectolin Suspension (attapulgite)	Y	L1
Pepto Bismol Caplets/Chewable Tablets/Liquid/Liquid Max (bismuth subsalicylate)	N	L3
Rheaban Tablets (attapulgite)	Y	L1

Y   *Usually safe when breastfeeding*

Y1   *Usually safe when breastfeeding (use of loperamide should not exceed more than two days)*

N   *Avoid when breastfeeding*

31

Artificial Sweeteners

Equal (aspartame)	Y1	L1
Neotame (acesulfame potassium)	Y	L1
NutraSweet (aspartame)	Y1	L1
Splenda (sucralose)	Y	L2
Stevia In The Raw (stevia extract)	Y	L3
SugarTwin (aspartame)	Y1	L1
Sunett (acesulfame potassium)	Y	L1
Sweet One (acesulfame potassium)	Y	L1
Sweet'N Low (saccharin)	Y	L3

Y *Usually safe when breastfeeding*

Y1 *Usually safe when breastfeeding (avoid using if mother or infant has been diagnosed with phenylketonuria)*

Asthma Preparations

Asthma Mist Inhaler (herbs)	Ø	L4
Asthmahaler Mist Inhaler (epinephrine)	Ø	L1
Asthmanephrin (Mist Inhaler (epinephrine)	Ø	L1
Bronkaid Mist Inhaler (epinephrine)	Ø	L1
Bronkaid Caplets (ephedrine/guaifenesin)	Ø	L4
Bronkotabs (ephedrine/guaifenesin)	Ø	L4
Primatene Mist Inhaler (epinephrine)	Ø	L1
Primatene Tablets (ephedrine/guaifenesin)	Ø	L4
Respitrol Liquid (herbs)	Ø	L4

Ø   *Consultation with a physician is highly recommended prior to use*

33

Callus, Corn, and Wart Products

Akurza (salicylic acid)	Y1	L2
Compound W (salicylic acid)	Y1	L2
Dr. Scholl's Callus Remover/Corn Remover/Corn and Callus Remover (salicylic acid)	Y1	L2
Dr. Scholl's Clear Away Wart Remover (salicylic acid)	Y1	L2
Dr. Scholl's Freeze Away (dimethyl ether/propane)	Y1	L2
Durasal Solution (salicylic acid)	Y1	L2
Duofilm (salicylic acid)	Y1	L2
Duoplant Corn Remover (salicylic acid)	Y1	L2
Freezone Wart Treatment (salicylic acid)	Y1	L2
Gordofilm Wart Remover Solution (salicylic acid)	Y1	L2
Hydrisalic Gel (salicylic acid)	Y1	L2
Keralyt Gel (salicylic acid)	Y1	L2
Mosco Callus & Corn Remover Liquid (salicylic acid)	Y1	L2
Occlusal-HP (salicylic acid)	Y1	L2
Panscol (salicylic acid)	Y1	L2
SalAcid Plasters (salicylic acid)	Y1	L2
Salactic Film (salicylic acid)	Y1	L2
Salicylic Acid Film/Gel/Liquid/Solution (salicylic acid)	Y1	L2
Sal-Plant Gel (salicylic acid)	Y1	L2
Tinamed Wart Remover (salicylic acid)	Y1	L2
Wartner Freezing Wart Remover (dimethyl ether/propane)	Y1	L2
Wart-Off Liquid (salicylic acid)	Y1	L2

Y1   Usually safe when breastfeeding (avoid breathing fumes)

Cold, Flu, and Allergy Products

Actifed Cold & Allergy Tablets (chlorpheniramine/phenylephrine)	Y1, Y2, Y3	L3
Advil Allergy Sinus Caplets (chlorpheniramine/ibuprofen/pseudoephedrine)	Y1, Y2, Y3	L3
Advil Cold & Sinus Caplets/Cold & Sinus Liqui-Gels (ibuprofen/pseudoephedrine)	Y2, Y3	L3
Alavert Oral Disintegrating Tablets/24-Hour Allergy Tablets (loratadine)	Y1, Y4	L1
Alavert D-12 Hour Allergy and Sinus Tablets (loratadine/pseudoephedrine)	Y1, Y2, Y3, Y4	L3
Aleve-D Cold & Sinus Caplets/Sinus & Headache Caplets (naproxen/pseudoephedrine)	Y2, Y3	L3
Alka-Seltzer Plus Day Cold Liquid Gels (acetaminophen/dextromethorphan/phenylephrine)	Y1, Y2, Y3	L3
Alka-Seltzer Plus Cold & Cough Liquid Gels/Plus Cold & Cough Liquid (acetaminophen/chlorpheniramine/dextromethorphan/phenylephrine)	Y1, Y2, Y3	L3
Alka-Seltzer Plus Cold Original Effervescent Tablets (aspirin/chlorpheniramine/phenylephrine)	N	L4
Alka-Seltzer Plus Flu Effervescent Tablets (aspirin/chlorpheniramine/dextromethorphan)	N	L4
Alka-Seltzer Plus Day & Night Cold Formula Effervescent Tablets/Plus Night Cold Formula Effervescent Tablets (aspirin/dextromethorphan/doxylamine/phenylephrine)	N	L4
Alka-Seltzer Plus Day & Night Liquid Gels/Plus Night Cold Formula Liquid Gels/Plus Night Cold Liquid (acetaminophen/dextromethorphan/doxylamine/phenylephrine)	Y1, Y2, Y3	L3

Alka-Seltzer Plus Mucus & Congestion Effervescent Tablets (dextromethorphan/guaifenesin)	Y1, Y3	L2
Alka-Seltzer Plus Sinus Formula Effervescent Tablets (aspirin/phenylephrine)	N	L4
Allerest Maximum Strength Tablets (chlorpheniramine/pseudoephedrine)	Y1, Y2, Y3	L3
Allerest No Drowsiness Allergy & Sinus Caplets (acetaminophen/pseudoephedrine)	Y2, Y3	L3
Allerest PE Allergy & Sinus Relief Tablets (chlorpheniramine/phenylephrine)	Y1, Y2, Y3	L3
Benadryl Allergy Kapgels/Allergy Quick Dissolve Strips/Allergy Ultratabs/Liqui-Gels (diphenhydramine)	Y1	L2
Benadryl Allergy & Sinus Kapgels/Allergy & Sinus Headache Kapgels/Severe Allergy & Sinus Headache Caplets (acetaminophen/diphenhydramine/phenylephrine)	Y1, Y2, Y3	L3
Benadryl Severe Allergy & Sinus Headache Caplets (acetaminophen/diphenhydramine/phenylephrine)	Y1, Y2, Y3	L3
Benadryl-D Allergy & Sinus Tablets (diphenhydramine/phenylephrine)	Y1, Y2, Y3	L3
Benylin Adult Formula Cough Syrup (dextromethorphan)	Y1	L1
Benylin All-In-One Cold & Flu Syrup/Cold & Sinus Rapid-Gels (acetaminophen/dextromethorphan/guaifenesin/pseudoephedrine)	Y1, Y2, Y3	L3
Benylin All-In-One Cold & Flu Nighttime Syrup (acetaminophen/chlorpheniramine/ dextromethorphan/guaifenesin/pseudoephedrine)	Y, Y2, Y3	L3
Benylin Chest Coughs Non-Drowsy Cough Syrup (guaifenesin/menthol)	Y1, Y3	L2
Benylin Cold & Sinus Plus Caplets/Cold & Sinus Tablets (acetaminophen/phenylephrine)	Y2, Y3	L3
Benylin DM Dry Cough Syrup (dextromethorphan)	Y1	L1

36

Benylin DM-D-E Chest Cough & Cold Syrup (dextromethorphan/guaifenesin/pseudoephedrine)	Y1, Y2, Y3	L3
Benylin DM-E Chest Cough Syrup/DM-E Chest Cough & Cold Syrup (dextromethorphan/guaifenesin)	Y1, Y3	L2
Benylin E Chest Congestion Syrup (guaifenesin/menthol)	Y1, Y3	L2
Benylin Extra Strength Cough & Cold Syrup (dextromethorphan/guaifenesin/menthol/pseudoephedrine)	Y1, Y2, Y3	L3
Buckley's Cough Mixture (dextromethorphan)	Y1	L1
Cheracol-D Syrup (dextromethorphan/guaifenesin)	Y1, Y3	L2
Chlor-Trimeton 4-Hour Allergy Tablets/Redi-Tabs (chlorpheniramine)	Y1	L3
Claritin 24 Hour Allergy Tablets (loratadine)	Y1, Y4	L1
Claritin-D 12 Hour Allergy & Congestion Tablets/24 Hour Allergy & Congestion Tablets (loratadine/pseudoephedrine)	Y1, Y2, Y3, Y4	L3
Comtrex Day & Night Severe Cold & Sinus Caplets (acetaminophen/chlorpheniramine/phenylephrine)	Y1, Y2, Y3	L3
Comtrex Deep Chest Cold Caplets (acetaminophen/guaifenesin)	Y3	L2
Comtrex Non-Drowsy Cold & Cough Caplets (acetaminophen/phenylephrine)	Y2, Y3	L3
Contact Cold & Flu Day & Night Caplets/Cold & Flu Maximum Strength Caplets (acetaminophen/chlorpheniramine/ phenylephrine)	Y1, Y2, Y3	L3
Contac Cold & Flu Non-Drowsy Maximum Strength Caplets (acetaminophen/phenylephrine)	Y2, Y3	L3
Coricidin HBP Chest Congestion & Cough Softgels (dextromethorphan/guaifenesin)	Y1, Y3	L2
Coricidin HBP Cough & Cold Tablets (chlorpheniramine/dextromethorphan)	Y1, Y3	L3

Coricidin HBP Cold & Flu Tablets (acetaminophen/ chlorpheniramine)	Y1, Y3	L3
Coricidin HPB Day-Night Multi-Symptom Tablets (acetaminophen/chlorpheniramine/guaifenesin/ dextromethorphan)	Y1, Y3	L3
Coricidin HBP Maximum Strength Flu Tablets (acetaminophen/chlorpheniramine/dextromethorphan)	Y1, Y2, Y3	L3
Coricidin HPB Nighttime Multi-Symptom Cold Relief Liquid (acetaminophen/dextromethorphan/doxylamine)	Y1, Y3	L3
Delsym 12 Hour Cough Relief Liquid (dextromethorphan)	Y1, Y4	L1
Dimetapp Cough & Cold Long-Acting Liquid (chlorpheniramine/dextromethorphan)	Y1, Y3, Y4	L3
Dimetapp Elixir Cold & Allergy (brompheniramine/ phenylephrine)	Y1, Y2, Y3	L3
Dimetapp Nighttime Cold & Congestion Liquid (diphenhydramine/phenylephrine)	Y1, Y2, Y3	L3
Dristan Cold Multi-Symptom Tablets (acetaminophen/ chlorpheniramine/phenylephrine)	Y1, Y2, Y3	L3
Drixoral 12 Hour Cold & Allergy Tablets (dexbrompheniramine/pseudoephedrine)	Y1, Y2, Y3, Y4	L3
Efidac 24 Chlorpheniramine Tablets (chlorpheniramine)	Y1, Y4	L3
Efidac 24 Capsules (pseudoephedrine)	Y2, Y4	L3
Efidac 24 (R) Capsules (chlorpheniramine/ pseudoephedrine)	Y1, Y2, Y3, Y4	L3
Excedrin Sinus Headache Caplets (acetaminophen/ phenylephrine)	Y2, Y3	L3

Guaifed Capsules (guaifenesin/phenylephrine)	Y2, Y3	L3
Guaitab Tablets (guaifenesin/pseudoephedrine)	Y2, Y3	L3
Humbid Capsules (guaifenesin)	Y	L2
Humbid E Oral Tablets (guaifenesin)	Y	L2
Humbid LA Capsules (guaifenesin)	Y4	L2
Humbid DM Sustained-Release Capsules (dextromethorphan/guaifenesin/potassium guaiacolsulfonate)	Y1, Y3, Y4	L2
Hyland's Cough Syrup (herbs)	N	L4
Hyland's C-Plus Cold Tablets (herbs/potassium iodide)	N	L5
Motrin IB Sinus Tablets (ibuprofen/pseudoephedrine)	Y2, Y3	L3
Mucinex Cold Mixed Berry Liquid (guaifenesin/ phenylephrine)	Y2, Y3	L2
Mucinex Cough Orange Crème Mini-Melts (dextromethorphan/guaifenesin)	Y1, Y3	L3
Mucinex Maximum Strength Tablets/Tablets (guaifenesin)	Y	L2
Mucinex D Extended-Release Tablets (guaifenesin/ pseudoephedrine)	Y2, Y3, Y4	L3
Mucinex DM Extended Release Tablets (dextromethorphan/guaifenesin)	Y1, Y2, Y4	L2
Novahistine Elixir (chlorpheniramine/phenylephrine)	Y1, Y2, Y3	L3
Novahistine DMX Elixir (dextromethorphan/ guaifenesin/pseudoephedrine)	Y1, Y2, Y3	L3
Oscillococcinum Pellets (Muscovy Duck Liver and Heart Extract)	N	L4
Pertussin DM Extra Strength Cough Syrup (dextromethorphan)	Y1	L1

Refenesen Chest Congestion Relief Caplets (guaifenesin)	Y	L2
Refenesen Chest Congestion & Pain Relief Caplets (acetaminophen/guaifenesin)	Y3	L2
Refenesen Chest Congestion & Pain Relief PE Caplets (acetaminophen/guaifenesin/phenylephrine)	Y2, Y3	L3
Robitussin Chest Congestion Liquid (guaifenesin)	Y	L2
Robitussin Cough & Chest Congestion DM Liquid/Cough & Chest Congestion DM Max Liquid/Cough & Chest Congestion Sugar-Free DM Liquid (guaifenesin/dextromethorphan)	Y1, Y3	L2
Robitussin Cough & Cold Long-Acting Liquid (chlorpheniramine/dextromethorphan)	Y1, Y3, Y4	L3
Robitussin Cough Long-Acting Liquid/CoughGels Liqui-Gels (dextromethorphan)	Y1, Y3, Y4	L1
Robitussin Cough & Cold CF Liquid (dextromethorphan/guaifenesin/phenylephrine)	Y1, Y2, Y3	L3
Robitussin Cough & Cold D Liquid (dextromethorphan/guaifenesin/pseudoephedrine)	Y1, Y2, Y3	L3
Robitussin Night Time Cough & Cold Liquid (diphenhydramine/phenylephrine)	Y1, Y2, Y3	L3
Robitussin Night Time Cough, Cold & Flu Liquid (acetaminophen/chlorpheniramine/dextromethorphan/phenylephrine)	Y1, Y2, Y3	L3
Scot-Tussin Diabetes CF Sugar-Free Liquid (dextromethorphan)	Y	L1
Scot-Tussin DM (chlorpheniramine/dextromethorphan)	Y1, Y2	L3
Scot-Tussin DM Maximum Strength Sugar-Free Liquid (chlorpheniramine/dextromethorphan)	Y1, Y3	L3
Scot-Tussin Original Sugar-Free Liquid (caffeine/pheniramine/phenylephrine/sodium salicylate)	N	L4
Scot-Tussin Senior Sugar-Free Liquid (dextromethorphan/guaifenesin)	Y1, Y3	L2

Silphen Cough Syrup, Old Formula (dextromethorphan)	Y1	L1
Simply Cough Liquid (dextromethorphan)	Y1	L1
Simply Stuffy Liquid (pseudoephedrine)	Y2	L3
Sinarest Drops (acetaminophen/chlorpheniramine/pseudoephedrine)	Y1, Y2, Y3	L3
Sinarest Syrup (acetaminophen/chlorpheniramine/menthol/pseudoephedrine/sodium citrate)	Y1, Y2, Y3	L3
Sinarest Tablets (acetaminophen/caffeine/chlorpheniramine)	Y1, Y3	L3
Sine-Aid Maximum Strength Tablets (acetaminophen/pseudoephedrine)	Y2, Y3	L3
Sine-Aid IB Tablets (ibuprofen/pseudoephedrine)	Y2, Y3	L3
Sine-Off Multi Symptom Relief Cold Cough Medicine Tablets/Strong, Fast Relief Sinus Cold Medicine Caplets (acetaminophen/chlorpheniramine/phenylephrine)	Y1, Y2, Y3	L3
Sine-Off Multi Symptom Relief Severe Cold Medicine Tablets (acetaminophen/guaifenesin/phenylephrine)	Y2, Y3	L3
Sine-Off Non-Drowsy Relief Maximum Strength Caplets (acetaminophen/phenylephrine)	Y2, Y3	L3
Sinutab Sinus Caplets (acetaminophen/phenylephrine)	Y2, Y3	L3
Sudafed Maximum Strength Sinus & Allergy Tablets (chlorpheniramine/phenylephrine)	Y1, Y2, Y3	L3
Sudafed Nasal Decongestant Tablets/PE Nasal Decongestant Tablets (pseudoephedrine)	Y2, Y4	L3
Sudafed Nasal 12-Hour Tablets/Nasal 24-Hour Tablets (pseudoephedrine)	Y2	L3
Sudafed PE Cold & Cough Caplets (acetaminophen/dextromethorphan/guaifenesin)	Y1, Y3	L3
Sudafed PE Nighttime Cold Caplets/PE Severe Cold Formula Caplets (acetaminophen/diphenhydramine/phenylephrine)	Y1, Y2, Y3	L3

Sudafed PE Nighttime Nasal Decongestant Tablets (diphenhydramine/phenylephrine)	Y1, Y2, Y3	L3
Sudafed PE Non-Drying Sinus Caplets (guaifenesin/phenylephrine)	Y2, Y3	L3
Sudafed PE Sinus & Allergy Tablets (chlorpheniramine/pseudoephedrine)	Y1, Y2, Y3	L3
Sudafed PE Sinus Headache Caplets (acetaminophen/phenylephrine)	Y2, Y3	L3
Sudafed PE Tablets (phenylephrine)	Y2	L3
Tavist Allergy 12-Hour Relief Tablets (clemastine)	N	L4
Theraflu Cold & Chest Warming Relief Liquid (acetaminophen/guaifenesin/phenylephrine)	Y2, Y3	L3
Theraflu Cold & Cough Hot Liquid (chlorpheniramine/dextromethorphan/phenylephrine)	Y1, Y2, Y3	L3
Theraflu Cold & Sore Throat Hot Liquid/Flu & Sore Throat Hot Liquid (acetaminophen/pheniramine/phenylephrine)	Y1, Y2, Y3	L3
Theraflu Daytime Severe Cold & Cough Caplets/Daytime Severe Cold & Cough Hot Liquid (acetaminophen/dextromethorphan/phenylephrine)	Y1, Y2, Y3	L3
Theraflu Flu & Chest Congestion Hot Liquid (acetaminophen/guaifenesin)	Y3	L2
Theraflu Flu & Sore Throat Relief Syrup/Nighttime Severe Cold & Cough Hot Liquid/Nighttime Warming Relief Syrup/Sugar-Free Nighttime Severe Cold & Cough Hot Liquid (acetaminophen/diphenhydramine/phenylephrine)	Y1, Y2, Y3	L3
Theraflu Nighttime Cold & Cough Thin Strips (diphenhydramine/phenylephrine)	Y1, Y2, Y3	L3
Theraflu Nighttime Severe Cold & Cough Caplets (acetaminophen/chlorpheniramine/dextromethorphan/phenylephrine)	Y1, Y2, Y3	L3
Triaminic Chest & Nasal Congestion Syrup (guaifenesin/phenylephrine)	Y2, Y3	L3

Triaminic Cold & Allergy Liquid (chlorpheniramine/phenylephrine)	Y1, Y2, Y3	L3
Triaminic Cold with Stuffy Nose Thin Strips (phenylephrine)	Y2, Y3	L3
Triaminic Cough and Runny Nose Softchews (chlorpheniramine/dextromethorphan)	Y1, Y3	L3
Triaminic Cough & Sore Throat Liquid/Cough & Sore Throat Softchews (acetaminophen/dextromethorphan)	Y1, Y3	L1
Triaminic D Multisymptom Cold Liquid (chlorpheniramine/dextromethorphan/pseudoephedrine)	Y1, Y2, Y3	L3
Triaminic Day Time Cold & Cough Liquid (dextromethorphan/phenylephrine)	Y1, Y2, Y3	L3
Triaminic Long-Acting Cough Liquid/Long Acting Cough Thin Strips (dextromethorphan)	Y1, Y4	L1
Triaminic Multisymptom Fever Liquid (acetaminophen/chlorpheniramine/dextromethorphan)	Y1, Y3	L3
Triaminic Nighttime Cold & Cough Liquid/Nighttime Cold & Cough Thin Strips (diphenhydramine/phenylephrine)	Y1, Y2, Y3	L3
Tylenol Allergy Complete Multi-Symptom Cool Burst Caplets (acetaminophen/chlorpheniramine/phenylephrine)	Y1, Y2, Y3	L3
Tylenol Allergy Complete Nighttime Cool Burst Caplets (acetaminophen/diphenhydramine/phenylephrine)	Y1, Y2, Y3	L3
Tylenol Allergy Multi-Symptom Nighttime Cool Burst Caplets/Allergy Multi-Symptom Rapid-Release Cool Burst Caplets/Allergy Multi-Symptom Rapid-Release Gelcaps/Sinus Congestion & Pain Nighttime Caplets (acetaminophen/chlorpheniramine/phenylephrine)	Y1, Y2, Y3	L3
Tylenol Cold Head Congestion Day-Night Pack Caplets/Cold Head Congestion Nighttime Caplets/Cold Multi-Symptom Day-Night Pack Caplets/Cold Multi-Symptom Nighttime Cool Burst Caplets (acetaminophen/chlorpheniramine/dextromethorphan/phenylephrine)	Y1, Y2, Y3	L3

Tylenol Cold Head Congestion Daytime Capsules/Cold Multi-Symptom Daytime Citrus Burst Liquid/Cold Multi-Symptom Daytime Rapid-Release Cool Burst Caplets/Cold Multi-Symptom Rapid-Release Gelcaps (acetaminophen/dextromethorphan/phenylephrine)	Y1, Y2, Y3	L3
Tylenol Cold Multi-Symptom Nighttime Cool Burst Liquid (acetaminophen/dextromethorphan/doxylamine/ phenylephrine)	Y1, Y2, Y3	L3
Tylenol Cold Multi-Symptom Severe Cool Burst Caplets/Cold Multi-Symptom Severe Cool Burst Liquid/Cold Severe Head Congestion Caplets (acetaminophen/dextromethorphan/phenylephrine)	Y1, Y2, Y3	L3
Tylenol Cough & Sore Throat Daytime Liquid (acetaminophen/dextromethorphan)	Y1, Y3	L1
Tylenol Cough & Sore Throat Nighttime Cool Burst-Honey Lemon Warming Liquid (acetaminophen/ dextromethorphan/doxylamine)	Y1, Y3	L3
Tylenol Severe Allergy Caplets (acetaminophen/ diphenhydramine)	Y1, Y3	L2
Tylenol Sinus Congestion & Pain Daytime Cool Burst Caplets/Sinus Congestion & Pain Daytime Gelcaps/Sinus Congestion & Pain Daytime Rapid-Release Gelcaps (acetaminophen/phenylephrine)	Y2, Y3	L3
Tylenol Sinus Congestion & Pain Nighttime Gelcaps (acetaminophen/chlorpheniramine/phenylephrine)	Y1, Y2, Y3	L3
Tylenol Sinus Congestion & Severe Pain Cool Burst Caplets (acetaminophen/guaifenesin/phenylephrine)	Y2, Y3	L3
Tylenol Sinus Severe Congestion Daytime Cool Burst Caplets (acetaminophen/guaifenesin/pseudoephedrine)	Y2, Y3	L3
Vicks DayQuil Cold & Flu Relief Liquicaps/DayQuil Cold & Flu Relief Liquid (acetaminophen/ dextromethorphan/phenylephrine)	Y1, Y2, Y3	L3
Vicks DayQuil Cough Liquid (dextromethorphan)	Y1	L1
Vicks DayQuil Sinus Liquicaps (acetaminophen/ phenylephrine)	Y2, Y3	L1
Vicks Formula 44 Custom Care Chesty Cough Liquid (dextromethorphan/guaifenesin)	Y1, Y3	L2

Vicks Formula 44 Custom Care Congestion Liquid (dextromethorphan/phenylephrine)	Y1, Y2, Y3	L3
Vicks Formula 44 Custom Care Cough & Cold PM Liquid (acetaminophen/chlorpheniramine/ dextromethorphan)	Y1, Y3	L3
Vicks Formula 44 Custom Care Dry Cough Suppressant Liquid (dextromethorphan)	Y1	L1
Vicks NyQuil Cold & Relief Liquicaps/NyQuil Cold & Flu Relief Liquid (acetaminophen/dextromethorphan/ doxylamine)	Y1, Y3	L3
Vicks NyQuil Cough Liquid (dextromethorphan/ doxylamine)	Y1, Y3	L3
Vicks NyQuil D Liquid (acetaminophen/ dextromethorphan/doxylamine/pseudoephedrine)	Y1, Y2, Y3	L3
Vicks Nyquil Sinus Liquicaps (acetaminophen/ doxylamine/phenylephrine)	Y1, Y2, Y3	L3
Zyrtec Tablets (cetirizine)	Y1	L2
Zyrtec-D Tablets (cetirizine/pseudoephedrine)	Y1, Y2, Y3	L3

Note: If decongestant is pseudoephedrine, occasional or short-term use is compatible during early stage breastfeeding with good milk production. Avoid in mothers with poor milk supply, especially six months after birth.

Note: Because of new Federal regulations controlling the sale of OTC pseudoephedrine products, some manufacturers have substituted phenylephrine for pseudoephedrine. Check labels carefully.

Y   *Usually safe when breastfeeding*
Y1   *Usually safe when breastfeeding (monitor infant for drowsiness and/ or excitability)*
Y2   *Usually safe when breastfeeding (monitor for decreased milk production; mother should drink extra fluids)*
Y3   *Usually safe when breastfeeding (best taken as individual ingredients to treat only specific symptoms)*
Y4   *Avoid long-acting dosage forms if possible*
N   *Avoid when breastfeeding*

Cough and Cold Inhalers, Lozenges, Rubs, and Sprays

Benzedrex Inhaler (propylhexedrine)	N	L4
Celestial Seasonings Soothers Herbal Throat Drops (herbs/menthol/pectin)	Y	L2
Cepacol Sore Throat Lozenges/Sore Throat Spray (benzocaine/menthol)	Y	L2
Cepastat Sore Throat Lozenges (eucalyptus/menthol/ phenol)	N	L4
Cheracol Sore Throat Spray (phenol)	N	L4
Chloraseptic Sore Throat Spray (phenol)	N	L4
Chloraseptic Sore Throat Lozenges (benzocaine/menthol)	Y	L2
Halls Cough Drops (eucalyptus/menthol)	Y	L2
HOLD Lozenges (dextromethorphan)	Y1	L1
N'ICE Lozenges (menthol)	Y	L1
Robitussin Sugar Free Throat Drops/Cough Drops (menthol)	Y	L1
Sucrets Complete Lozenges (dyclonine/menthol/pectin/ vitamin C/zinc)	Y	L3
Sucrets DM Cough Formula Lozenges (dextromethorphan)	Y1	L1
Sucrets Herbal Lozenges (herbs/menthol/pectin/ vitamin C)	Y	L3
Sucrets ICE (echinacea/menthol/pectin/zinc)	Y	L1
Sucrets Sore Throat Lozenges (dyclonine)	Y	L3
Theraflu Vapor Patch (camphor/eucalyptus/menthol)	Y	L2
Triaminic Vapor Patch Cough (camphor/menthol)	Y	L2
Vicks Cough Drops (menthol)	Y	L1
Vicks Formula 44 Custom Care Sore Throat Lozenges (benzocaine/menthol)	Y	L2
Vicks VapoInhaler (levmetamfetamine)	Y1	L3

Vicks VapoRub Cream/Ointment (camphor/eucalyptus/menthol)	Y	L2
Vicks VapoSteam (camphor)	Y	L2

Y   *Usually safe when breastfeeding*
Y1   *Usually safe when breastfeeding (monitor infant for drowsiness and/ or excitability)*
N   *Avoid when breastfeeding*

Dandruff, Psoriasis, and Seborrhea Treatments

Dandrex Shampoo (selenium sulfide)	Y	L3
Denorex Dandruff Daily Protection Shampoo (pyrithione zinc)	Y	L2
Denorex Dandruff Extra Strength Shampoo (salicylic acid)	Y	L2
Denorex Therapeutic Protection Shampoo/Therapeutic Protection 2-in-1 Shampoo (coal tar)	Y	L3
Dermarest Psoriasis Medicated Moisturizer/Psoriasis Medicated Overnight Treatment/Psoriasis Medicated Skin Treatment/Psoriasis Scalp Treatment/Psoriasis Medicated Shampoo-Conditioner (salicylic acid)	Y	L2
DHS SAL Shampoo (salicylic acid)	Y	L2
DHS Tar Dermatological Hair & Scalp Shampoo/Tar Gel Shampoo/Tar Shampoo (coal tar)	Y	L3
DHS Zinc Shampoo (pyrithione zinc)	Y	L2
Head & Shoulders Citrus Breeze Dandruff Conditioner/Citrus Breeze Dandruff Shampoo Plus Conditioner/Citrus Breeze Dandruff Shampoo (pyrithione zinc)	Y	L2
Head & Shoulders Classic Clean Dandruff Conditioner/Classic Clean Dandruff Shampoo Plus Conditioner/Classic Clean Dandruff Shampoo (pyrithione zinc)	Y	L2
Head & Shoulders Dandruff Intensive Treatment Shampoo (selenium sulfide)	Y	L3
Head & Shoulders Dry Scalp Care Dandruff Conditioner/Dry Scalp Care Dandruff Shampoo Plus Conditioner/Dry Scalp Care Dandruff Shampoo (pyrithione zinc)	Y	L2
Head & Shoulders Extra Volume Dandruff Shampoo (pyrithione zinc)	Y	L2

Head & Shoulders Intensive Treatment Shampoo (selenium sulfide)	Y	L3
Head & Shoulders Ocean Lift Shampoo Plus Dandruff Conditioner/Ocean Lift Dandruff Shampoo (pyrithione zinc)	Y	L2
Head & Shoulders Refresh Dandruff Shampoo Plus Conditioner/Refresh Dandruff Shampoo (pyrithione zinc)	Y	L2
Head & Shoulders Restoring Shine Dandruff Shampoo Plus Conditioner/Restoring Shine Dandruff Shampoo (pyrithione zinc)	Y	L2
Head & Shoulders Sensitive Care Dandruff Shampoo Plus Conditioner/Sensitive Care Dandruff Shampoo (pyrithione zinc)	Y	L2
Head & Shoulders Smooth & Silky Dandruff Conditioner/Smooth & Silky Dandruff Shampoo Plus Conditioner/Smooth & Silky Dandruff Shampoo (pyrithione zinc)	Y	L2
Ionil Plus Conditioning Shampoo (salicylic acid)	Y	L2
Ionil-T Plus Shampoo/Shampoo (coal tar)	Y	L3
L'Oreal Homme Purete Anti-Dandruff Shampoo (pyrithione zinc)	Y	L2
MG217 Ointment/Medicated Lotion/Tar Shampoo (coal tar)	Y	L3
Neutrogena T-Gel Daily Control Dandruff Shampoo (pyrithione zinc)	Y	L2
Neutrogena T-Gel Daily Control 2-in-1 Dandruff Shampoo Plus Conditioner (pyrithione zinc)	Y	L2
Neutrogena T-Gel Extra Strength Shampoo/Original Formula Shampoo/Stubborn Itch Control Shampoo (coal tar)	Y	L3
Neutrogena T/Sal Therapeutic Conditioner/Scalp Build-Up Control Shampoo (salicylic acid)	Y	L2
Nizoral Anti-Dandruff Shampoo (ketoconazole)	Y	L2
P&S Liquid/Shampoo (glycerin/mineral oil)	Y	L1
Pantene Pro-V Anti-Dandruff Shampoo + Conditioner (pyrithione zinc)	Y	L2

Pert Plus Dandruff Control Shampoo Plus Conditioner/ 2-in-1 Dandruff Dismissed Shampoo (pyrithione zinc)	Y	L2
Psoriasin Gel/Liquid Dab-On/Ointment (coal tar)	Y	L3
Psoriasin Therapeutic Shampoo and Body Wash (salicylic acid)	Y	L2
Scalpicin Anti-Itch Liquid Scalp Treatment (salicylic acid)	Y	L2
Scalpicin Maximum Strength Liquid (hydrocortisone)	Y	L2
Sebex Shampoo (salicylic acid/sulfur)	Y	L2
Sebulex Medicated Dandruff Shampoo (salicylic acid/ sulfur)	Y	L2
Selsun Blue Dandruff Shampoo/Dandruff Shampoo Plus Conditioner/Medicated Treatment Dandruff Shampoo/Moisturizing Formula Dandruff Shampoo/Normal to Oily Formula Dandruff Shampoo/ 2-in-1 Dandruff Shampoo (selenium sulfide)	Y	L3
Selsun Blue Naturals Dandruff Shampoo (salicylic acid)	Y	L2
Selsun Salon Shampoo Plus Conditioner (pyrithione zinc)	Y	L2
Selsun Salon 2-in-1 Pyrithione Zinc Shampoo (pyrithione zinc)	Y	L2
Suave Dandruff Control Shampoo (sulfur)	Y	L2
Zincon Medicated Dandruff Shampoo (pyrithione zinc)	Y	L2
ZNP Shampoo Bar (pyrithione zinc)	Y	L2

Y   Usually safe when breastfeeding

Heart Attack and Stroke Risk Reduction Agents

Anacin 81 Tablets (81 mg aspirin)	Y	L3
Aspirin Tablets (81 mg)	Y	L3
Bayer Low Dose Aspirin Chewable Tablets/Low Dose Aspirin Safety Coated Tablets (81 mg aspirin)	Y	L3
Bayer Women's Low Dose Aspirin Caplets (81 mg aspirin/calcium carbonate)	Y	L3
Ecotrin Low Strength Tablets (81 mg aspirin)	Y	L3
Halfprin 81 mg Tablets (81 mg aspirin)	Y	L3
Halfprin 162 mg Tablets (162 mg aspirin)	Y	L3
Healthprin Adult Low Strength Aspirin Tablets (81 mg aspirin)	Y	L3
Healthprin Half Dose Aspirin Tablets (162.5 mg aspirin)	Y	L3
St. Joseph Chewable Aspirin Tablets/Enteric Safety-Coated Tablets (81 mg aspirin)	Y	L3

Y   *Usually safe when breastfeeding*

Hemorrhoidal Preparations

Americaine Hemorrhoidal Ointment (benzocaine)	Y	L2
Anusol HC Ointment/Suppositories (hydrocortisone)	Y	L2
Balneol Hygienic Cleansing Lotion (lanolin oil/mineral oil/moisturizers)	Y	L1
Calmol 4 Hemorrhoidal Suppositories (cocoa butter/zinc oxide)	Y	L1
Citrucel Caplets/Powder (methylcellulose)	Y	L1
Colace Capsules/Liquid/Syrup (docusate sodium)	Y	L2
Docusol Constipation Relief Mini Enemas (docusate sodium)	Y	L2
Dulcolax Stool Softener Capsules (docusate sodium)	Y	L2
Equalactin Chewable Tablets (calcium polycarbophil)	Y	L1
Fibercon Caplets (calcium polycarbophil)	Y	L1
Fleet Sof-Lax Tablets (docusate)	Y	L2
Hemspray Hemorrhoidal Relief Spray (camphor/glycerin/phenylephrine/witch hazel)	Y	L3
Kaopectate Liqui-Gels (docusate calcium)	Y	L2
Konsyl Easy Mix Powder/Orange Powder/Original Powder (psyllium)	Y	L1
Konsyl-D Powder (psyllium)	Y	L1
Metamucil Capsules/Original Texture Powder/Smooth Texture Powder-Orange/Wafers (psyllium)	Y	L1
Nupercainal Cream/Ointment (dibucaine)	Y	L3
Peterson's Ointment (methysalicylate)	Y	L3
Phillips Stool Softener Capsules (docusate sodium)	Y	L2
Preparation H Anti-Itch Cream (hydrocortisone)	Y	L2
Preparation H Hemorrhoidal Cooling Gel (phenylephrine/witch hazel)	Y	L3
Preparation H Hemorrhoidal Cream Maximum Strength Pain Relief (glycerin/phenylephrine/pramoxine/white petrolatum)	Y	L3

Preparation H Hemorrhoidal Ointment (mineral oil/ petrolatum/phenylephrine/shark liver oil)	Y	L3
Preparation H Hemorrhoidal Suppositories (cocoa butter/ phenylephrine/shark liver oil)	Y	L3
Preparation H Medicated Wipes (witch hazel)	Y	L1
Procto Foam Spray (pramoxine)	Y	L1
Procto Foam-HC Spray (hydrocortisone/pramoxine)	Y	L2
Rectacaine Hemorrhoidal Ointment (dibucaine)	Y	L3
T.N. Dickinson's Witch Hazel Hemorrhoidal Pads (witch hazel)	Y	L1
Tronolane Anesthetic Hemorrhoidal Cream (pramoxine/ zinc oxide)	Y	L1
Tronolane Cream (pramoxine)	Y	L1
Tronolane Suppositories (hard fat/phenylephrine)	Y	L3
Tucks Anti-Itch Ointment (hydrocortisone)	Y	L2
Tucks Hemorrhoidal Ointment (mineral oil/pramoxine/ zinc oxide)	Y	L1
Tucks Medicated Pads/Take Alongs Medicated Towelettes (witch hazel)	Y	L1
Tucks Topical Starch Hemorrhoidal Suppositories (topical starch)	Y	L1
Wyanoids-HC Rectal Suppositories (belladonna/ bismuth/boric acid/ephedrine/hydrocortisone/Peruvian balsam/zinc oxide)	N	L4

Y   *Usually safe when breastfeeding*
N   *Avoid when breastfeeding*

Insulin Preparations

All insulin preparations are safe for use during breastfeeding; however, it is recommended that the insulin dose be reduced, with the concurrence of the patient's physician, by 25% of the prepregnancy dose	Y	L1
Glutose 15/Glutose 45 (oral glucose gel for treatment of insulin reaction)	Y	L1

Note: Insulin is not sold over-the-counter (OTC) in all States of the USA

Y   *Usually safe when breastfeeding*

Laxatives and Stool Softeners

Alophyn Enteric Coated Stimulant Laxative Pills (bisacodyl)	Y1	L2
Benefiber Powder/Stick Packs Powder (natural fiber)	Y	L1
Benefiber Plus Calcium Powder (calcium/natural fiber)	Y	L1
Bisacodyl Tablets (bisacodyl)	Y1	L2
Carters Laxative Sodium Free Pills (bisacodyl)	Y1	L2
Cascara Sagrada Tablets (cascara sagrada)	Y1	L3
Castor Oil	N	L3
Ceo-Two Evacuant Suppositories (potassium bitartrate/ sodium bicarbonate)	Y	L2
Citrucel Caplets/Powder (methylcellulose)	Y	L1
Colace Capsules/Liquid/Syrup (docusate sodium)	Y	L2
Colace Glycerin Suppositories for Adults and Children (glycerin)	Y	L2
Correctol Tablets (bisacodyl)	Y1	L2
Docusol Constipation Relief Mini Enemas (docusate sodium)	Y	L2
Doxidan Tablets (bisacodyl)	Y1	L2
Dulcolax Stool Softener Capsules (docusate sodium)	Y	L2
Dulcolax Suppositories/Tablets (bisacodyl)	Y1	L2
Epsom Salts (magnesium sulfate)	Y	L1
Equalactin Chewable Tablets (calcium polycarbophil)	Y	L1
Evac-Q-Kwik Bowel Cleansing System (bisacodyl/saline)	Y1	L2
Ex-Lax Maximum Strength Tablets/Tablets (sennosides)	Y1	L3
Ex-Lax Ultra Stimulant Laxative Tablets (bisacodyl)	Y1	L2
Fiberall Powder (psyllium)	Y	L1
Fibercon Tablets (calcium polycarbophil)	Y	L1
Fleet Bisacodyl Enema/Suppositories (bisacodyl)	Y1	L2

Fleet Enema/Enema Extra (monobasic-dibasic sodium phosphate)	Y	L1
Fleet Mineral Oil Enema (mineral oil)	Y	L1
Fleet Sof-Lax Softgels (docusate)	Y	L1
Fleet Stimulant Laxative Tablets (sennosides)	Y1	L3
Glycerin Suppositories (glycerin)	Y	L1
Herb-Lax Tablets (herbs/senna)	Y1	L3
Hydrocil Instant Fiber Laxative Powder (psyllium)	Y	L1
Innerclean Herbal Blend/Herbal Tablets (herbs/psyllium/senna)	Y1	L3
Kaopectate Liqui-Gels (docusate calcium)	Y	L1
Kellogg's Castor Oil (castor oil)	N	L3
Kondremul Emulsion (mineral oil)	Y	L1
Konsyl Easy Mix Powder/Orange Powder/Original Powder (psyllium)	Y	L1
Konsyl Fiber Caplets (calcium polycarbophil)	Y	L1
Konsyl Senna Prompt Capsules (psyllium/sennosides)	Y1	L3
Magnesium Citrate Solution (magnesium citrate)	Y1	L1
Konsyl-D Powder (psyllium)	Y	L1
Maltsupex Liquid (malt soup extract powder/potassium sorbate/sodium propionate)	Y	L1
Metamucil Capsules/Original Texture Powder-Orange/Smooth Texture Powder-Orange/Wafers (psyllium)	Y	L1
Perdiem Overnight Relief Tablets (sennosides)	Y1	L3
Peri-Colace Tablets (docusate/sennosides)	Y1	L3
Phillips Antacid/Laxative Chewable Tablets/Milk of Magnesia Concentrated Liquid/Milk of Magnesia Liquid (magnesium hydroxide)	Y	L1
Phillips M-O Liquid (magnesium hydroxide/mineral oil)	Y	L1
Phillips Cramp-Free Laxative Caplets (magnesium)	Y1	L1
Phillips Stool Softener Capsules (docusate sodium)	Y	L1
Regu-Lax Drops (picosulphate)	Y1	L3
Regu-Lax Forte Tablets (herbs)	N	L4

56

Regu-Lax Tablets (herbs/rhubarb/senna)	N	L4
Senokot Tablets/XTRA Tablets (sennosides)	Y1	L3
Senokot S Tablets (docusate/sennosides)	Y1	L3
Serutan Granules (psyllium)	Y	L1
Surfak Liqui-Gels (calcium docusate)	Y	L2

Y   *Usually safe when breastfeeding*
Y1   *Usually safe when breastfeeding (do not use for more than one or two doses)*
N   *Avoid when breastfeeding*

Nasal Preparations

Afrin No Drip All Night 12 Hour Pump Mist/No Drip Extra Moisturizing Nasal Spray/No Drip Original Pump Mist Nasal Spray/No Drip Severe Congestion Nasal Spray/No Drip Sinus Nasal Spray (oxymetazoline)	Y1	L3
Alconefrin Nasal Drops (phenylephrine)	Y1	L3
Allergy Buster Nasal Spray (capsaicin/nettle)	Y	L3
Ayr Allergy & Sinus Nasal Mist/Saline Nasal Mist (sodium chloride)	Y	L1
Ayr Saline Nasal Gel No-Drip Sinus Spray (aloe/glycerin/sodium chloride starch)	Y	L1
Ayr Saline Nasal Gel With Soothing Aloe (aloe/dimethicone/glycerin/sodium chloride)	Y	L1
Dristan Nasal Spray (phenylephrine/pheniramine)	Y1	L3
Dristan 12 Hour Nasal Spray (oxymetazoline)	Y1	L3
ENTSOL Buffered Hypertonic Nasal Irrigation Mist/Buffered Hypertonic Saline Nasal Spray (sodium chloride)	Y1	L1
ENTSOL Nasal Gel with Aloe and Vitamin E (aloe/dimethicone/glycerin/sodium chloride/vitamin E)	Y1	L1
Duration 12 Hour Spray (oxymetazoline)	Y1	L3
4-Way Fast Acting Nasal Decongestant Spray (phenylephrine)	Y1	L3
4-Way Mentholated Nasal Decongestant Spray (menthol/phenylephrine)	Y1	L3
4-Way Saline Moisturizing Mist (boric acid/eucalyptol/glycerin/menthol/sodium chloride)	Y	L2
Intal Inhaler (cromolyn sodium)	Y	L1
Mucinex Full Force Nasal Spray (oxymetazoline)	Y1	L3
Nasal Comfort (aloe/sodium chloride)	Y	L1
NasalCrom Nasal Allergy Symptom Prevention and Controller Nasal Spray (cromolyn sodium)	Y	L1
Nasal Moist Nasal Gel/Nasal Spray (aloe/sodium chloride)	Y	L1

Neo-Synephrine Extra Strength Nasal Spray/Mild Formula Nasal Spray/Nighttime Nasal Spray (phenylephrine)	Y1	L3
Nose Better Natural Mist Moisturizing Spray (glycerin/sodium chloride)	Y	L1
Nose Better Non-Greasy Aromatic Relief Gel (eucalyptol/menthol)	Y	L2
Nostrilla Complete Congestion Relief Nasal Spray/Original Fast Relief Nasal Spray (oxymetazoline)	Y1	L3
Nostrilla Conditioning Double Moisture Nasal Spray (povidone/sodium chloride/spearmint oil/wintergreen oil)	N	L2
Ocean Premium Saline Nasal Spray (sodium chloride)	Y	L1
Otrivin Nasal Drops/Nasal Spray (xylometazoline)	Y1	L3
Pretz Moisturizing Nasal Spray (glycerin/sodium chloride)	Y	L1
Privine Nasal Spray (naphazoline)	Y1	L3
Salinex Nasal Lubricant/Nasal Spray (sodium chloride)	Y	L1
Similasan Hay Fever Relief Non-Drowsy Formula Nasal Spray (herbs)	N	L4
Simply Saline Sterile Saline Nasal Mist (sodium chloride)	Y1	L1
Sinarest Nasal Spray (oxymetazoline)	Y1	L3
SinoFresh Nasal & Sinus Care Spray (eucalyptus oil/peppermint oil sodium chloride/wintergreen oil)	Y	L2
Sinus Buster Nasal Spray (capsaicin)	Y	L3
Sudafed OM Sinus Cold Nasal Spray/OM Sinus Congestion Nasal Spray (oxymetazoline)	Y1	L3
Sudafed Sinus Cold 12 Hour Nasal Spray/Sinus Congestion 12 Hour Nasal Spray (oxymetazoline)	Y1	L3
Triaminic Decongestant Spray Nasal & Sinus Congestion (xylometazoline)	Y1	L3
Vicks Sinex Nasal Spray For Sinus Relief (phenylephrine)	Y1	L3
Vicks Sinex 12 Hour Nasal Spray/12 Hour Ultra Fine Mist for Sinus Relief (oxymetazoline)	Y1	L3
Zicam Allergy Relief Nasal Gel (herbs/sulfur)	N	L4
Zicam Allergy Relief Homeopathic Nasal Solution Pump (herbs/sulfur)	N	L4

Zicam Allergy Relief with Cooling Menthol Gel Swabs (herbs/menthol)	N	L4
Zicam Extreme Congestion Relief Liquid Nasal Spray/Intense Sinus Relief Liquid Nasal Spray (oxymetazoline)	Y1	L3
Zicam No-Drip Liquid Nasal Gel (zincum gluconicum)	N	L4
Zicam Sinus Relief Liquid Nasal Gel (aloe/eucalyptus/ glycerin/menthol)	Y	L2

Y   *Usually safe when breastfeeding*
Y1   *Usually safe when breastfeeding (monitor for decreased milk production; mother should drink extra fluids)*
N   *Avoid when breastfeeding*

Nausea, Vomiting, and Motion Sickness Products

Benadryl Capsules/Liquid/Tablets (diphenhydramine)	Y1	L2
Bonine Chewable Tablets (meclizine)	Y1	L3
Calm-X Tablets (dimenhydrinate)	Y1	L2
Dramamine Chewable Tablets/Original Tablets (dimenhydrinate)	Y1	L2
Dramamine Less Drowsy Formula Tablets (meclizine)	Y1	L3
Emetrol Cherry Syrup (phosphorated carbohydrates)	Y	L1
Humco Cola Syrup (cola syrup)	Y	L1
Pepto Bismol Caplets/Chewable Tablets/Liquid/Liquid Max (bismuth subsalicylate)	N	L3
Marezine For Motion Sickness Tablets (cyclizine)	Y1	L3
Nauzene Chewable Tablets (diphenhydramine)	Y1	L2
Triptone For Motion Sickness Tablets (dimenhydrinate)	Y1	L2

Y   *Usually safe when breastfeeding*

Y1   *Usually safe when breastfeeding (monitor infant for drowsiness and/ or excitability)*

N   *Avoid when breastfeeding*

Ophthalmics (Eye Medicines)

AK-Nefrin Eye Drops (phenylephrine)	Y	L3
Akwa Tears Lubricant Eye Drops (benzalkonium/ polyvinyl alcohol)	Y	L1
Akwa Tears Lubricant Ophthalmic Ointment (lanolin/ mineral oil/white petrolatum)	Y	L1
Alaway Eye Drops (kerotifen)	Y	L2
Allergan Lacri-Lube S.O.P. Lubricant Eye Ointment (mineral oil/white petrolatum)	Y	L1
Allergan Relief Redness Reliever & Lubricant Eye Drops (phenylephrine/polyvinyl alcohol)	Y	L3
Allerest Eye Drops (naphazoline)	Y	L3
Allergy Eye Drops (naphazoline)	Y	L3
Allersol Eye Drops (naphazoline)	Y	L3
AMO Blink Tears Lubricating Eye Drops for Mild-Moderate Dry Eyes (polyethylene glycol 400)	Y	L1
Artelac Eye Drops (hypromellose)	Y	L1
Bausch & Lomb Advanced Eye Relief Redness Maximum Relief (hypromellose/naphazoline)	Y	L3
Bausch & Lomb Advanced Eye Relief Dry Eye Environmental Lubricant Eye Drops (glycerin)	Y	L1
Bausch & Lomb Advanced Eye Relief Dry Eye Rejuvenation Lubricant Eye Drops (glycerin/propylene glycol)	Y	L1
Bausch & Lomb Advanced Eye Relief Night Time Lubricant Eye Ointment Preservative Free (mineral oil/ white petrolatum)	Y	L1
Bausch & Lomb Eye Wash (irrigating solution)	Y	L1
Bausch & Lomb Moisture Eyes PM (mineral oil/white petrolatum)	Y	L1
Bausch & Lomb Soothe Lubricant Eye Drops (glycerin/ propylene glycol)	Y	L1

Bion Tears Lubricant Eye Drops (dextran/hydroxypropyl methylcellulose)	Y	L1
Claritin Eye Drops (ketotifen)	Y	L2
Clear Eyes ACR Seasonal Relief (glycerin/naphazoline/zinc sulfate)	Y	L3
Clear Eyes for Dry Eyes (carboxymethylcellulose/glycerin)	Y	L1
Clear Eyes Redness Relief (glycerin/naphazoline)	Y	L3
Collyrium for Fresh Eyes Eye Wash (borate solution)	Y	L1
Comfort Eye Drops (naphazoline)	Y	L3
Degest2 Eye Drops (naphazoline)	Y	L3
Eye Allergy Relief Eye Drops (naphazoline/pheniramine)	Y	L3
Eyelube Ointment (hypromellose)	Y	L1
GenTeal Gel/Mild Dry Eyes Drops/Moderate Dry Eyes Drops (hypromellose)	Y	L1
GenTeal Lubricant Eye Drops for Moderate to Severe Dry Eye Relief Gel Drops (carboxymethylcellulose/hypromellose)	Y	L1
GenTeal PM Ointment (mineral oil/white petrolatum)	Y	L1
Gonak Eye Drops (hypromellose)	Y	L1
Goniosoft Eye Drops (hypromellose)	Y	L1
Goniovisc Eye Drops (hypromellose)	Y	L1
Hypo Tears/HypoTears PF (polyethylene glycol 400/polyvinyl alcohol)	Y	L1
Hypo Tears Ointment (mineral oil/white petrolatum)	Y	L1
Hypo Tears Plus (polyethylene glycol 400/polyvinyl alcohol/povidone)	Y	L1
Isopto Tears (hypromellose)	Y	L1
Just Tears (hypromellose)	Y	L1
Lubri-Tears Lubricant Eye Ointment (lanolin/mineral oil/white petrolatum)	Y	L1
Murine Tears Lubricant Eye Drops (polyvinyl alcohol/povidone)	Y	L1
Murine Tears Plus Eye Drops (dextran/polyvinyl alcohol/povidone/tetrahydrozoline)	Y	L3

Muro 128 Ointment/Solution (sodium chloride)	Y	L1
Naphazoline Plus Eye Drops (naphazoline/pheniramine)	Y	L3
Naphcon Eye Drops (naphazoline)	Y	L3
Naphcon-A Eye Drops (naphazoline/pheniramine)	Y	L3
Nature's Tears (hypromellose)	Y	L1
Ocucoat Eye Drops/Ocucoat PF Eye Drops (hypromellose)	Y	L1
Oculotect Eye Drops (povidone)	Y	L1
Ocu-Tears (hypromellose)	Y	L1
Opcon-A Allergy Relief Drops (naphazoline/pheniramine)	Y	L3
Opcon-A Eye Drops (antazoline/naphazoline)	Y	L3
Opticrom Allergy Eye Drops (cromolyn sodium)	Y	L1
Opti-Clear Eyewash (buffered isotonic salt solution)	Y	L1
Opti-Clear Redness Reliever Eye Drops (tetrahydrozoline)	Y	L3
Optics Laboratory Minidrops Eye Therapy (polyvinyl alcohol/polyvinylpyrrolidone)	Y	L1
Refresh Celluvisc (carboxymethylcellulose)	Y	L1
Refresh Classic (carboxymethylcellulose)	Y	L1
Refresh Eye Itch Relief (ketotifen)	Y	L2
Refresh Lacri-Lube (carboxymethylcellulose)	Y	L1
Refresh Liquigel (carboxymethylcellulose)	Y	L1
Refresh Optive/Optive Sensitive (carboxymethylcellulose)	Y	L1
Refresh Plus (carboxymethylcellulose)	Y	L1
Refresh P.M. (mineral oil/white petrolatum)	Y	L1
Refresh Tears (carboxymethylcellulose)	Y	L1
Relief Eye Drops (phenylephrine)	Y	L3
Rohto V Arctic Eye Drops (hypromellose/tetrahydrozoline)	Y	L3
Rohto V Cool Redness Relief Drops (naphazoline/polysorbate 80)	Y	L3
Rohto V Ice Eye Drops (hypromellose/tetrahydrozoline/zinc sulfate)	Y	L3
Rohto Zi For Eyes Lubricant Eye Drops (povidone)	Y	L1

Similasan Dry Eye Relief Eye Drops (herbs)	N	L4
Similasan Pink Eye Relief Eye Drops (herbs)	N	L4
Similasan Stye Eye Relief Eye Drops (herbs)	N	L4
Soothe Lubricant Eye Drops (glycerin/propylene glycol)	Y	L1
Soothe XP Emollient Lubricant Eye Drops (light mineral oil/mineral oil)	Y	L1
Steri-Optics Eyewash (buffered isotonic salt solution)	Y	L1
Systane Liquid Gel Drops/Lubricant Eye Drops/Preservative Free Lubricant Eye Drops/Ultra Lubricant Eye Drops (polyethylene glycol 400/propylene glycol)	Y	L1
Systane Nighttime Lubricant Eye Ointment (mineral oil/ white petrolatum)	Y	L1
Tearisol Eye Drops (hypromellose)	Y	L1
Tears Again Eye Drops/Liquid Gel Drops (hypromellose)	Y	L1
Tears Again Eye Ointment (mineral oil/white petrolatum)	Y	L1
Tears Naturale Forte Lubricant Eye Drops (dextran/ glycerin/hypromellose)	Y	L1
Tears Naturale Free Lubricant Eye Drops/II Polyquad Lubricant Eye Drops (dextran/hypromellose)	Y	L1
Tears Naturale P.M. Lubricant Eye Ointment (mineral oil/ white petrolatum)	Y	L1
Tetrasine Eye Drops (tetrahydrozoline)	Y	L1
TheraTears Liquid Gel Lubricant Eye Gel/Lubricant Eye Drops (carboxymethylcellulose)	Y	L1
Ultra Tears (hypromellose)	Y	L1
VasoClear Eye Drops (naphazoline)	Y	L3
VasoClear-A Eye Drops (naphazoline)	Y	L3
Vasocon A Eye Drops (antazoline/naphazoline)	Y	L3
Visine-A Eye Drops (naphazoline/pheniramine)	Y	L3
Visine A.C. Astringent Redness Reliever Drops (tetrahydrozoline/zinc sulfate)	Y	L3
Visine Advanced Redness Reliever & Lubricant Drops (dextran/polyethylene glycol 400/povidone/ tetrahydrozoline)	Y	L3

Visine Allergy Relief Drops/Original Drops/Moisturizing Drops (tetrahydrozoline)	Y	L3
Visine L.R. Redness Reliever Drops (oxymetazoline)	Y	L3
Visine Maximum Redness Relief (glycerin/hypromellose/ propylene glycol 400/tetrahydrozoline)	Y	L3
Visine Multi-Symptom Relief (glycerin/hypromellose/ propylene glycol 400/tetrahydrozoline/zinc sulfate)	Y	L3
Visine Pure Tears Lubricant Eye Drops (glycerin/ hypromellose/polyethylene glycol 400)	Y	L1
Visine Tired Eye Relief (glycerin/hypromellose/ polyethylene glycol 400)	Y	L1
Visine Total Eye Soothing Wipes (cleansing agents/water)	Y	L1
Viva-Drops (polysorbate 80)	Y	L1
Zaditor Eye Drops (ketotifen)	Y	L2
Zincfrin Eye Drops (phenylephrine)	Y	L3
Zyrtec Itchy Eye Drops (ketotifen)	Y	L2

Y   *Usually safe when breastfeeding*
N   *Avoid when breastfeeding*

Oral Hygiene Products

Abreva Cold Sore/Fever Blister Treatment/Pump Cold Sore/Fever Blister Treatment (docosanol)	Y	L2
Act Mouthwash (sodium fluoride)	Y2	L2
Aim Toothpaste (sodium fluoride)	Y1	L2
Amosan Oral Wound Cleanser Powder Packs (sodium perborate monohydrate)	Y	L1
Anbesol Cold Sore Therapy Ointment (allantoin/benzocaine/camphor white petrolatum/vitamin E)	Y	L2
Anbesol Gel/Liquid (allantoin/benzocaine/camphor)	Y	L2
Anbesol Regular Strength Gel/Regular Strength Liquid/Maximum Strength Gel/Maximum Strength Liquid (benzocaine)	Y	L2
Anti-Plaque Dental Rinse (alcohol/benzoic acid/glycerin/sorbitol/tetrasodium pyrophosphate)	Y2	L2
Aquafresh Toothpaste (sodium fluoride)	Y1	L2
Aquafresh Sensitive Toothpaste (fluoride/potassium nitrate)	Y1	L3
Aquafresh White Trays (hydrogen peroxide)	Y	L1
Arm & Hammer Toothpaste (baking soda/sodium fluoride)	Y1	L2
Benzodent Cream (benzocaine)	Y	L2
Campho-Phenique Cold Sore Gel (camphor/phenol)	N	L4
Chloraseptic Pocket Pump Sore Throat Spray (phenol)	N	L4
Close-Up Mouthwash (sodium fluoride)	Y2	L2
Close-Up Toothpaste (sodium fluoride)	Y1	L2
Colgate Toothpaste (sodium fluoride)	Y1	L2
Colgate Simply White Gel (carbamide peroxide)	Y	L1
Crest Toothpaste (sodium fluoride)	Y1	L2
Crest Toothpaste (baking soda/peroxide/sodium fluoride)	Y1	L2
Crest Sensitivity Toothpaste (sodium fluoride/potassium nitrate)	Y1	L2

Crest Whitestrips (hydrogen peroxide)	Y	L1
Dr. Snapz Swabplus Mouth Sore Relief Swabs (benzocaine)	Y	L2
Fluorigard Rinse (sodium fluoride)	Y2	L2
Gly-Oxide Liquid (carbamide peroxide)	Y	L1
Hydrogen Peroxide Rinse (hydrogen peroxide)	Y	L1
Herpecin-L Lip Balm Stick (dimethicone)	Y	L2
Kank-A Mouth Pain Liquid (benzocaine/compound benzoin tincture)	Y	L3
Kank-A Soft Brush Tooth Mouth Pain Gel/Soothing Beads (benzocaine)	Y	L2
Mentadent Toothpaste (sodium fluoride)	Y1	L2
Mentadent Toothpaste (baking soda/peroxide/sodium fluoride)	Y1	L2
Novitra Cold Sore Maximum Strength Cream (zincum oxydatum)	N	L4
Oral Balance Gel/Liquid (bio-enzymes)	Y	L2
Orabase with Benzocaine Gel/Paste (benzocaine)	Y	L2
Orajel Antiseptic Mouth Sore Rinse (hydrogen peroxide)	Y	L1
Orajel Medicated Mouth Cold Sore Brush (allantoin/benzocaine/dimethicone/white petrolatum)	Y	L2
Orajel Ultra Mouth Sore Medicine Film-Forming Gel (benzocaine/menthol)	Y	L2
Orajel Medicated Mouth Sore Swabs/Protective Mouth Sore Discs (benzocaine)	Y	L2
Orajel Mouth Sore Medicine Gel (benzocaine/benzalkonium-zinc chloride)	Y	L3
Pepsodent Powder/Toothpaste (sodium fluoride)	Y1	L2
Pepsodent Toothpaste (baking powder/sodium fluoride)	Y1	L2
Peroxyl Rinse (hydrogen peroxide)	Y	L1
Phos Flur Rinse (sodium fluoride)	Y2	L2
Plax Rinse (alcohol/benzoic acid/glycerin/sorbitol/tetrasodium pyrophosphate)	Y2	L2
Releev 1-Day Cold Sore Treatment (benzalkonium chloride)	Y	L3

Rembrandt Canker Sore Toothpaste (citroxain/peroxide/ sodium fluoride)	Y1	L2
Rembrandt Toothpaste (citroxain/peroxide/sodium fluoride)	Y1	L2
Rembrandt Whitening Gel/Whitening Strips (hydrogen peroxide)	Y	L2
Rincinol P.R.N. Rinse (sodium hyaluronate)	Y	L1
Sensodyne Toothpaste (fluoride/potassium nitrate)	Y1	L2
Swab Plus Swabs (aluminum trihydroxide/magnesium peroxide)	Y	L1
Ultra Brite Toothpaste (sodium fluoride)	Y1	L2
Ultra Brite Toothpaste (baking soda/peroxide/sodium fluoride)	Y1	L2
Zilactin-B Canker Sore Gel/Long Lasting Mouth Sore Gel/6 Hour Canker & Mouth Sore Relief Gel (benzocaine)	Y	L2
Zilactin Early Relief Cold Sore Gel/Tooth and Gum Instant Pain Reliever (benzyl alcohol)	Y	L2
Zilactin -L Cold Sore Early Relief Liquid (lidocaine)	Y	L2
Zilactin Lip Balm (dimethicone/menthol)	Y	L1
Mouthwashes (Non-Fluoride): Biotene, Cepacol, Crest Pro Health, Listerine, Mentadent, Oasis, Scope, Smart Mouth, Store Brands, Tom's of Maine, (alcohol/ benzalkonium chloride/calcium/cetylpyridinium/ enzymes/eucalyptol/hexetidine/hydrogen peroxide/ menthol/methylsalicylate/sodium saccharin/thymol/ water)	Y3	L2

Y   *Usually safe when breastfeeding*

Y1 *Usually safe when breastfeeding (do not use if sodium fluoride exceeds 0.243% or fluoride ion exceeds 0.16% w/v)*

Y2 *Usually safe when breastfeeding (do not use if sodium fluoride exceeds 5 mg/10 ml; do not swallow after using)*

Y3 *Usually safe when breastfeeding (do not swallow after using)*

N   *Avoid when breastfeeding*

Otics (Ear Medications)

Acetic Acid Otic Solution (acetic acid)	Y	L1
Auralgan Ear Drops (benzocaine/glycerol/phenazone)	Y	L2
Auro Ear Drops (carbamide peroxide)	Y	L1
Auro-Dri Ear Drying Aid (glycerin/isopropyl alcohol)	Y	L1
Debrox Ear Drops (carbamide peroxide)	Y	L1
Hyland's Earache Drops (herbs)	Y	L3
Mack's Dry-n-Clear Ear Drying Aid (glycerin/isopropyl alcohol)	Y	L1
Murine Ear Wax Removal System (carbamide peroxide)	Y	L1
Physicians' Choice Ear Wax Removal Kit (carbamide peroxide)	Y	L1
ProEar Ear Drops (plant extracts)	Y	L3
Similasan Ear Wax Relief Ear Drops (glycerin)	Y	L1
Swim Ear Drying Aid (glycerin/isopropyl alcohol)	Y	L1
Traumeel Ear Drops (herbs)	Y	L3

Y   *Usually safe when breastfeeding*
N   *Avoid when breastfeeding*

Pediculosis (Lice) Treatments

G.B.H. Shampoo (lindane)	N	L4
Kewll Shampoo (lindane)	N	L4
Lice Freee! Gel (natrum muriaticum)	Y	L3
LiceMD Liquid (dimethicone)	Y	L1
Lice Shield Spray Shampoo (natural oil extracts)	Y	L1
Lindane Lotion/Shampoo (gamma-hexachlorocyclohexane)	N	L4
Nix Cream Rinse (permethrin)	Y	L2
Permethrin Lotion (permethrin)	Y	L2
RID Lotion/Spray (piperonyl butoxide/pyrethrum extract)	Y	L2
Rite Aid Lice Pyrinyl Shampoo (piperonyl butoxide)	Y	L2
Wild Child Quit Nits Cream/Spray (natural Australian ingredients)	Y	L3
Total Lice Shampoo (piperonyl butoxide/pyrethrum extract)	Y	L2

Y   *Usually safe when breastfeeding*
N   *Avoid when breastfeeding*

Pinworm Treatments

Pin-X Pinworm Treatment Suspension (pyrantel pamoate)	Y	L3
Pronto Plus Pinworm Treatment Suspension (pyrantel pamoate)	Y	L3
Reese's Pinworm Treatment Suspension/Tablets (pyrantel pamoate)	Y	L3

Y   *Usually safe when breastfeeding*

Skin Lubricants and Moisturizers

Alpha Keri Cream (vitamin E)	Y1	L1
Alpha Keri Original Lotion (sunflower oil/vitamin E)	Y1	L1
Alpha Keri Shower & Bath Oil (lanolin oil/mineral oil)	Y1	L1
Amlactin Moisturizing Cream/Lotion (lactic acid)	Y1	L1
Amlactin XL Moisturizing Lotion (ammonium-potassium-sodium lactate)	Y1	L1
Ammonium Lactate Lotion (ammonium lactate)	Y1	L1
Aqua Care Lotion (urea)	Y1	L1
Aquaphor Healing Ointment (glycerin/lanolin/mineral oil/petrolatum)	Y1	L1
Aquaphor Original Ointment (lanolin/mineral oil/petrolatum)	Y1	L1
Aveeno Bath Treatment (colloidal oatmeal)	Y1	L1
Aveeno Creamy Moisturizing Oil (dimethicone/glycerin)	Y1	L1
Aveeno Daily Moisturizer Ultra-Calming APF 15(dimethicone)	Y1	L1
Aveeno Daily Moisturizing Lotion (dimethicone)	Y1	L1
Aveeno Intense Relief Hand Cream (dimethicone)	Y1	L1
Aveeno Intense Relief Overnight Cream (dimethicone)	Y1	L1
Aveeno Moisturizing Bar for Dry Skin (dimethicone)	Y1	L1
Aveeno Moisturizing Lotion Skin Relief (dimethicone)	Y1	L1
Aveeno Positively Radiant Moisturizing Lotion (dimethicone/glycerin)	Y1	L1
Aveeno Positively Radiant Moisturizing Lotion SPF 15 (dimethicone)	Y1	L1
Aveeno Positively Smooth Moisturizing Lotion (dimethicone/glycerin)	Y1	L1
Aveeno Radiant Skin Daily Moisturizer with SPF 15 (dimethicone)	Y1	L1
Aveeno Skin Relief Body Wash Fragrant Free (glycerin)	Y1	L1

Aveeno Skin Relief Moisturizing Cream (dimethicone/ glycerin)	Y1	L1
Aveeno Ultra-Calming Night Cream (glycerin)	Y1	L1
Carmol-10 Cream (urea)	Y1	L1
Carmol-10 Lotion (urea)	Y1	L1
Cetaphil Daily Advance Ultra Hydrating Lotion (glycerin)	Y1	L1
Cetaphil Daily Facial Moisturizer SPF 15 with Parsol 1789 (glycerin)	Y1	L1
Cetaphil Moisturizing Cream (dimethicone/petrolatum)	Y1	L1
Cetaphil Moisturizing Lotion (dimethicone/glycerin)	Y1	L1
Cetaphil Therapeutic Hand Cream (glycerin)	Y1	L1
Cetaphil UVA-UVB Defense SPF 50 (dimethicone/ glycerin)	Y1	L1
Cocoa Butter Stick (cocoa butter)	Y1	L1
Corn Huskers Lotion (glycerin)	Y1	L1
Curel Continuous Comfort Fragrance Free Lotion (dimethicone/glycerin)	Y1	L1
Curel Continuous Comfort Original Formula Lotion (dimethicone/glycerin)	Y1	L1
Curel Natural Healing Soothing Lotion (glycerin)	Y1	L1
Curel Natural Healing Nourishing Lotion (glycerin)	Y1	L1
Curel Ultra Healing Intensive Moisture Lotion (glycerin)	Y1	L1
Eucerin Cream Original (lanolin/mineral oil/petrolatum)	Y1	L1
Eucerin Dry Skin Therapy Calming Cream (dimethicone/ glycerin)	Y1	L1
Eucerin Lotion Daily Replenishing (dimethicone/ glycerin/sunflower oil)	Y1	L1
Eucerin Lotion Original (lanolin/mineral oil)	Y1	L1
Eucerin Plus Intensive Repair Hand Cream (dimethicone/ glycerin/urea)	Y1	L1
Eucerin Plus Intensive Repair Lotion (glycerin/lanolin/ mineral oil)	Y1	L1
Eucerin Plus Smoothing Essentials (dimethicone/ dimethicone/urea)	Y1	L1

Eucerin Redness Relief Daily Perfecting Lotion SPF 15 (dimethicone/glycerin)	Y1	L1
Eucerin Redness Relief Soothing Cleanser (glycerin)	Y1	L1
Eucerin Redness Relief Soothing Moisture Lotion SPF 15 (dimethicone/glycerin)	Y1	L1
Eucerin Redness Relief Soothing Night Cream (dimethicone/glycerin)	Y1	L1
Eucerin Sensitive Facial Skin Gentle Hydrating Cleanser (glycerin/lanolin/mineral oil)	Y1	L1
Gold Bond Ultimate Comfort Body Powder (corn starch)	Y1	L1
Gold Bond Ultimate Healing Lotion (dimethicone/ glycerin/petrolatum)	Y1	L1
Johnson's Baby Oil (mineral oil)	Y1	L1
Johnson's Baby Powder (aloe/corn starch/vitamin E)	Y1	L1
Keri Age Defy & Protect Lotion (ammonium lactate/ glycerin/vitamin E)	Y1	L1
Keri Long Lasting Hand Cream (dimethicone/mineral oil/vitamin E)	Y1	L1
Keri Lotion Sensitive Skin (dimethicone/glycerin/ vitamin E)	Y1	L1
Keri Moisture Therapy Advance Extra Dry Skin Lotion (dimethicone/glycerin)	Y1	L1
Keri Nourishing Shea Butter Lotion (glycerin/mineral oil/ shea butter)	Y1	L1
Keri Original Formula Lotion (glycerin/mineral oil/ vitamin E)	Y1	L1
Keri Overnight Deep Conditioning Lotion (dimethicone/ glycerin)	Y1	L1
Keri Renewal Milk Body Lotion (dimethicone/sunflower oil)	Y1	L1
Keri Renewal Serum for Dry Skin (dimethicone/ sunflower oil)	Y1	L1
Lac-Hydrin Five Lotion (ammonium hydroxide/ dimethicone/lactic acid)	Y1	L1
Lanolin Ointment Hydrous (lanolin)	Y1	L1

Lubriderm Advanced Therapy Hand Cream (dimethicone/glycerin)	Y1	L1
Lubriderm Advanced Therapy Moisturizing Lotion (dimethicone/glycerin/mineral oil)	Y1	L1
Lubriderm Advanced Therapy Triple Smoothing Lotion (glycerin/petrolatum)	Y1	L1
Lubriderm Daily Moisture Fragrance Free Lotion (glycerin/mineral oil)	Y1	L1
Lubriderm Daily Moisture Lotion (glycerin/mineral oil)	Y1	L1
Lubriderm Daily Moisturizer Lotion SPF 15 (urea/ vitamin E/white petrolatum)	Y1	L1
Lubriderm Intense Skin Repair Body Cream (glycerin/ mineral oil/petrolatum)	Y1	L1
Lubriderm Intense Skin Repair Body Lotion (glycerin/ mineral oil/petrolatum)	Y1	L1
Lubriderm Intense Skin Repair Body Lotion with Itch Relief (dimethicone/glycerin/petrolatum)	Y1	L1
Lubriderm Sensitive Skin Therapy Moisturizing Lotion (glycerin/mineral oil/petrolatum)	Y1	L1
Lubriderm Skin Nourishing Moisturizing Lotion with Premium Oat Extract (glycerin/oat kernel extract)	Y1	L1
Lubriderm Skin Nourishing Moisturizing Lotion with Sea Kelp Extract (glycerin/giant kelp leaf extract/petrolatum)	Y1	L1
Lubriderm Skin Nourishing Moisturizing Lotion with Shea and Cocoa Butter (cocoa butter/dimethicone/ glycerin/shea butter)	Y1	L1
Mineral Oil	Y1	L1
Neutrogena Deep Moisture Body Cream (dimethicone/ glycerin)	Y1	L1
Neutrogena Norwegian Formula Body Moisturizer (dimethicone/glycerin/oatmeal)	Y1	L1
Neutrogena Norwegian Formula Deep Moisture Hand Cream (cocoa butter/glycerin/petrolatum)	Y1	L1
Neutrogena Norwegian Formula Hand Cream (glycerin)	Y1	L1
Nivea Body Age Defying Formula Deep Moisturizer For Body (dimethicone/glycerin/mineral oil)	Y1	L1

Nivea Cream (glycerin/lanolin/mineral oil/petrolatum)	Y1	L1
Nivea Body Original Moisture Daily Lotion Dry Skin (dimethicone/glycerin/lanolin/mineral oil)	Y1	L1
Nivea Essentially Enriched Lotion (mineral oil/ petrolatum)	Y1	L1
Nivea Smooth Sensation Body Oil (dimethicone/glycerin/ mineral oil)	Y1	L1
Nivea Smooth Sensation Daily Lotion Dry Skin (dimethicone/glycerin/lanolin/ mineral oil)	Y1	L1
Petroleum Jelly (white petrolatum)	Y1	L1
pHisoderm Cream Cleanser (aloe/chamomile/vitamin E)	Y1	L1
Pond's Cold Cream (mineral oil/sodium borate)	Y1	L1
Tuck's Medicated Cooling Pads (witch hazel)	Y1	L1
Vaseline Intensive Care Aloe Cool & Fresh Moisturizing Lotion (aloe/glycerin/lanolin/sunflower oil)	Y1	L1
Vaseline Intensive Care Cocoa Butter Deep Conditioning Lotion (cocoa butter/dimethicone/glycerin/vitamin E/ white petrolatum)	Y1	L1
Vaseline Intensive Care Healthy Hand & Nail Lotion (dimethicone/glycerin/vitamin E)	Y1	L1
Vaseline Intensive Care Lotion Total Moisture (glycerin/ petrolatum)	Y1	L1
Vaseline Intensive Rescue Clinical Therapy Lotion (dimethicone/glycerin/mineral oil)	Y1	L1
Vaseline Intensive Rescue Heal & Repair Balm (glycerin/ petrolatum)	Y1	L1
Vaseline Intensive Rescue Healing Hand Cream (dimethicone/glycerin/mineral oil/vitamin E)	Y1	L1
Vaseline Intensive Rescue Moisture Locking Butter (dimethicone/glycerin/petrolatum)	Y1	L1
Vaseline Intensive Rescue Moisture Locking Lotion (glycerin/petrolatum)	Y1	L1
Vaseline Jelly (white petrolatum)	Y1	L1
Vitamins A & D Ointment (cod liver oil/lanolin)	Y1	L1

Witch Hazel	Y1	L1
Zinc Oxide Ointment (zinc oxide)	Y1	L1

Note: Primary lubricating and cleansing agents are listed for each product. Even though similar products may contain the same primary ingredients, other ingredients may vary. Individual products may also contain acids, alcohols, animal by-products, dyes, emulsifiers, enzymes, fillers, food products, fragrances, herbs, minerals, moisturizers, oils, preservatives, stabilizers, sun screens, vitamins, and/or water. These ingredients are usually compatible with breastfeeding because they are applied topically in very low concentrations. Always check each individual product's ingredients to determine if they are the most suitable for your skin and that you are not allergic to any of the ingredients

Y1   *Usually safe when breastfeeding (if applied to nipple and/or areola, clean area with warm water and mild soap before breastfeeding)*

Sleep Aid Preparations

Advil PM Caplets/Liqui-Gels (diphenhydramine/ ibuprofen)	Y1, Y2	L2
Alka-Seltzer PM Effervescent Tablets (aspirin/ diphenhydramine)	N	L4
Anacin PM Aspirin Free Tablets (acetaminophen/ diphenhydramine)	Y1, Y2	L2
Bayer PM Caplets (aspirin/diphenhydramine)	N	L4
Benadryl Capsules (diphenhydramine)	Y1	L2
Compoz Gel Caps (diphenhydramine)	Y1	L2
Doan's Extra Strength PM Caplets (magnesium salicylate/diphenhydramine)	N	L4
Dormin Capsules (diphenhydramine)	Y1	L2
Excedrin PM Caplets/Tablets (acetaminophen/ diphenhydramine)	Y1, Y2	L2
Goody's PM Powders (acetaminophen/ diphenhydramine)	Y1, Y2	L2
Headache Relief PM Tablets (acetaminophen/ diphenhydramine)	Y1, Y2	L2
Hyland's Calms Forte Tablets (herbs/minerals)	N	L4
Hyland's Nerve Tonic (herbs)	N	L4
Legatrin PM Caplets (acetaminophen/ diphenhydramine)	Y1, Y2	L2
Mapap PM Caplets (acetaminophen/diphenhydramine)	Y1, Y2	L2
Melatonex Tablets (melatonin/vitamin B6)	Y3	L3
Melatonin Pills (melatonin)	Y3	L3
Midol PM Caplets/Maximum Strength Caplets/ Maximum Strength Menstrual Complete Caplets (acetaminophen/diphenhydramine)	Y1, Y2	L2
Mid Nite Chewable Tablets (chamomile/lemon/ melatonin)	Y1	L2

Mid Nite PM Chewable Tablets (bromelain/chamomile/ lemon/melatonin)	Y1	L2
Motrin PM Caplets (ibuprofen/diphenhydramine)	Y1, Y2	L2
Nytol Quick Caps Caplets/Quick Gels Capsules (diphenhydramine)	Y1	L2
Panadol Night Tablets (acetaminophen/ diphenhydramine)	Y1, Y2	L2
Simply Sleep Nighttime Sleep Aid Caplets (diphenhydramine)	Y1	L2
Sleep-Eze D Gelcaps (diphenhydramine)	Y1	L2
Sleep Rite Tablets (diphenhydramine)	Y1	L2
Sleepinal Capsules (diphenhydramine)	Y1	L2
Sominex Original Formula Tablets/Maximum Strength Formula Caplets (diphenhydramine)	Y1	L2
Tylenol PM Caplets/Geltabs/Rapid Release Gelcaps/ Vanilla Liquid (acetaminophen/diphenhydramine)	Y1, Y2	L2
Unisom Nighttime Sleep-Aid Sleep Tabs (doxylamine)	N	L4
Unisom Sleepmelts (diphenhydramine)	Y1	L2

Y1   *Usually safe when breastfeeding (monitor infant for drowsiness and/ or excitability)*

Y2   *Usually safe when breastfeeding (best taken as individual ingredients to treat only specific symptoms)*

Y3   *Usually safe when breastfeeding (total melatonin dose of 1 mg to 3 mg per day is acceptable)*

N   *Avoid when breastfeeding*

Smoking Cessation Aids

Commit Stop Smoking 2 mg Lozenges/Stop Smoking 4 mg Lozenges (nicotine polacrilex)	Y1	L3
Habitrol Nicotine Transdermal System Patch Step 1/Patch Step 2/Patch Step 3 (nicotine)	Y1	L3
Nica Patches (nicotine)	Y1	L3
Nicoderm CQ Step 1 Clear Patch/CQ Step 2 Clear Patch/CQ Step 3 Clear Patch (nicotine)	Y1	L3
Nicorelief Gum (nicotine polacrilex)	Y1	L3
Nicorette Gum/Lozenges/Mini Lozenges (nicotine polacrilex)	Y1	L3
Nicorrete Plus Gum (nicotine polacrilex)	Y1	L3
Nicorette 2 mg Patch/4 mg Patch (nicotine)	Y1	L3
Nicotine Gum (nicotine polacrilex)	Y1	L3
Nicotine Lozenges (nicotine polacrilex)	Y1	L3
Nicotine Transdermal System Patches (nicotine)	Y1	L3
Nicotrol Gum (nicotine polacrilex)	Y1	L3
Nicotrol Patches (nicotine)	Y1	L3
Thrive Gum (nicotine polacrilex)	Y1	L3

Y1 *Usually safe when breastfeeding (follow directions explicitly and do not smoke when using this product)*

Stimulants

No Doz Tablets (caffeine, 200 mg)	N1	L2
Vivarin Tablets (caffeine, 200 mg)	N1	L2

N1   Avoid when breastfeeding (less than 150 mg two to three times a day has no apparent effect on breastfeeding infant; probably better to drink a cup of coffee or tea or serving of soda than to take drug).

For caffeine content of beverages, please see the following tables:

COFFEE (5 oz cup)	CAFFEINE CONTENT (mg)
Drip method	110-150
Percolated	64-124
Instant	40-108
Decaffeinated	2-5
Instant Decaffeinated	2

TEA (5 oz cup)	CAFFEINE CONTENT (mg)
1 minute brew	9-33
3 minute brew	20-46
5 minute brew	20-50
Instant tea	12-28
Iced tea (12 oz cup)	22-36

SOFT DRINK/SODA (12 oz serving)	CAFFEINE CONTENT (mg)
Jolt	72.0
Sugar-Free Mr Pibb	58.8
Mountain Dew	54.0
Mello Yello	52.8
Tab	46.8
Coca-Cola	45.6
Coke	45.6
Diet Coke	45.6
Shasta Cola	44.4
Shasta Cherry Cola	44.4
Shasta Diet Cola	44.4
Shasta Diet Cherry Cola	44.4
Mr Pibb	40.8
Pibb Xtra	40.8
Dr Pepper	39.6
Big Red	38.4
Sugar-Free Dr Pepper	39.6
Pepsi-Cola	38.4
Aspen	36.0
Diet Pepsi	36.0
Pepsi Light	36.0
RC Cola	36.0
Diet Rite	36.0
Kick	31.2
Canada Dry Jamaica Cola	30.0
Canada Dry Diet Cola	1.2

Sunscreen Agents

Sunscreen Agent		Maximum % Concentration	
Aminobenzoic acid (PABA)	Y1	15	Y1
Avobenzone	Y1	3	Y1
Benzophenone-9	Y1	10	Y1
Cinoxate	Y1	3	Y1
Dioxybenzone	Y1	3	Y1
Ecamsule	Y1	3	Y1
Homosalate	Y1	15	Y1
Isopentenyl-4-methoxycinnamate	Y1	10	Y1
Methyl anthranilate	Y1	5	Y1
Methylbenzylidene camphor	Y1	4	Y1
Mexoryl XL	Y1	15	Y1
Neo Heliopan AP	Y1	10	Y1
Octocrylene	Y1	10	Y1
Octyl methoxycinnamate	Y1	7.5	Y1
Octyl salicylate	Y1	5	Y1
Oxybenzone	Y1	6	Y1
Padimate O	Y1	8	Y1
Parsol SLX	Y1	10	Y1
Phenylbenzimidazole sulfonic acid	Y1	4	Y1
Sulisobenzone	Y1	10	Y1
Tinosorb M	Y1	10	Y1
Tinosorb S	Y1	10	Y1
Titanium dioxide	Y1	25	Y1
Trolamine salicylate	Y1	12	Y1
Uvasorb HEB	Y1	10	Y1
Uvinul A Plus	Y1	10	Y1

Uvinul T 150	Y1	5	Y1
Zinc oxide	Y1	25	Y1

Y1   *Usually safe when breastfeeding (do not use sunscreen agents exceeding maximum % concentration; if applied to nipple and/ or areola, clean area with warm water and mild soap before breastfeeding)*

Topical Anti-Inflammatory and Anti-Itch Products

Product		
Aveeno Hydrocortisone 1% Anti-Itch Cream (hydrocortisone)	Y1	L2
Aveeno Anti-Itch Concentrated Lotion/Calamine & Pramoxine HCl Anti-Itch Cream (calamine/camphor/pramoxine hydrochloride)	Y2	L2
Aveeno Skin Relief Moisturizing Cream (dimethicone)	Y1	L1
Bactine Original First Aid Liquid/Pain Relieving Cleansing Spray (benzalkonium chloride/lidocaine)	Y2	L2
Benadryl Extra Strength Itch Stopping Cream/Extra Strength Itch Stopping Relief Stick/Extra Strength Spray/Original Strength Itch Stopping Cream (diphenhydramine HCl/zinc acetate)	Y2	L1
Benadryl Gel (diphenhydramine hydrochloride)	Y1	L1
Benadryl Itch Stopping Extra Strength Gel (diphenhydramine HCl)	Y1	L1
CalaGel Anti-Itch Gel (benzethonium chloride/diphenhydramine HCl/zinc acetate)	Y2	L2
Caladryl Anti-Itch Lotion (calamine/pramoxine)	Y2	L2
Caladryl Clear Anti-Itch Lotion (pramoxine/zinc acetate)	Y2	L2
Calamine Lotion (calamine/zinc oxide)	Y2	L2
Cortaid Advanced 12-Hour Anti-Itch Cream/Intensive Therapy Cooling Spray/Intensive Therapy Moisturizing Cream/Maximum Strength Cream/ Maximum Strength Ointment (hydrocortisone)	Y1	L2
Cortaid Poison Ivy Care Toxin Removal Cloths (citric acid/glycerin/hydantoin)	Y2	L1
Cortaid Poison Ivy Care Treatment Kit (pramoxine/zinc acetate)	Y2	L2
Corticool Gel (hydrocortisone)	Y1	L2

Cortizone-10 Cool Relief Gel/Creme/Creme Plus/Easy Relief Applicator/Intensive Healing Formula/Maximum Strength Anti-Itch Ointment/Ointment (hydrocortisone)	Y1	L2
Dermarest Eczema Medicated Lotion (hydrocortisone)	Y1	L2
Domeboro Astringent Solution Powder Packets (aluminum sulfate/calcium acetate)	Y2	L1
Gold Bond Extra Strength Medicated Body Lotion/Medicated Body Lotion (dimethicone/menthol)	Y2	L1
Gold Bond Medicated Extra Strength Powder/Medicated Powder (menthol/zinc oxide)	Y2	L2
Gold Bond Medicated Maximum Strength Anti-Itch Cream (menthol/pramoxine hydrochloride)	Y2	L2
Gold Bond Quick Spray (benzethonium chloride/menthol)	Y2	L2
Hydrocortisone Cream 0.5%/1% (hydrocortisone)	Y1	L2
Hydrocortisone Lotion 1% (hydrocortisone)	Y1	L2
Hydrocortisone Ointment 0.5%/1% (hydrocortisone)	Y1	L2
Ivarest Double Relief Formula (calamine/benzyl alcohol/diphenhydramine HCl)	Y2	L2
Ivy Block Lotion (bentoquatam)	Y2	L2
Ivy-Dry Anti-Itch Cream with Zytrel/Cream with Zytrel (camphor/menthol/zinc acetate)	Y2	L2
Ivy-Dry Scrub with Zytrel (allantoin/glycerin/zinc acetate)	Y2	L2
Ivy-Dry Super with Zytrel (benzyl alcohol/camphor/menthol/zinc acetate)	Y2	L2
Lanacaine Antibacterial First Aid Spray/Maximum Strength Cream/Original Strength Cream (benzethonium/benzocaine)	Y2	L2
Lanacaine Anti-Itch Ultra Moisturizing Maximum Strength Cream (benzethonium chloride/benzocaine)	Y2	L2
Sarna Sensitive Lotion (pramoxine)	Y2	L2
Sarna Ultra Anti-Itch Cream (menthol/pramoxine/white petrolatum)	Y2	L2
Solarcaine Aloe Extra Burn Relief Gel/Aloe Extra Burn Relief Spray (aloe/lidocaine)	Y2	L2

Solarcaine First Aid Medicated Spray (benzocaine/triclosan)	Y2	L2
Vaseline Intensive Rescue Clinical Therapy Lotion (dimethicone)	Y1	L1
Zinc Oxide Ointment (zinc oxide)	Y2	L2

Y1   *Usually safe when breastfeeding (if applied to nipple and/or areola, clean area with warm water and mild soap before breastfeeding)*

Y2   *Usually safe when breastfeeding (do not apply to breasts)*

Topical Antifungals

Clearly Confident Triple Action Fungus Treatment Cream (butenafine)	Y1	L2
Clotrimazole Cream (clotrimazole)	Y1	L1
Cruex Cream/Powder/Spray (undecylenic acid)	Y1	L2
Cruex Prescription Strength Cream/Lotion/Powder/Spray (miconazole)	Y1	L2
Desenex Antifungal Liquid Spray/Antifungal Powder/Antifungal Spray (miconazole)	Y1	L2
Desenex Cream (clotrimazole)	Y1	L1
FungiCure Anti-Fungal Gel (tolnaftate)	Y1	L2
FungiCure Anti-Fungal Liquid/Professional Formula Liquid (undecylenic acid)	Y1	L2
FungiCure Intensive Spray/Manicure-Pedicure Formula Liquid/Maximum Strength Anti-Fungal Liquid Spray (clotrimazole)	Y1	L1
Fungi Nail Anti-Fungal Solution (undecylenic acid)	Y1	L2
Gordochom Solution (chloroxylenol/undecylenic acid)	Y1	L2
Ketoconazole Cream (ketoconazole)	Y1	L2
Lamasil AT Continuous Spray/Cream/Gel (terbinafine)	Y1	L2
Lotrimin AF Antifungal Aerosol Liquid Spray/Antifungal Jock Itch Aerosol/ Antifungal Powder (miconazole)	Y1	L2
Lotrimin AF Antifungal Athlete's Foot Cream/For Her Antifungal Cream (clotrimazole)	Y1	L1
Micatin Cream (miconazole)	Y1	L2
Lotrimin Ultra Antifungal Cream (butenafine)	Y1	L2
Miconazole Cream (miconazole)	Y1	L2
Miracle of Aloe Miracure Anti-Fungal Liquid (aloe/tolnaftate)	Y1	L2
Neosporin AF Athlete's Foot Antifungal Spray Liquid/Athlete's Foot Antifungal Spray Powder/Athlete's Foot Cream/Jock Itch Antifungal Cream (miconazole)	Y1	L2

Nizoral Cream (ketoconazole)	Y1	L2
Tinactin Antifungal Absorbent Powder/Antifungal Cream/Antifungal Deodorant Powder Spray/Antifungal Jock Itch Powder Spray/Antifungal Liquid Spray/Antifungal Powder Spray (tolnaftate)	Y1	L2
Tineacide Antifungal Cream (undecylenic acid)	Y1	L2
Zeasorb Super Absorbent Antifungal Powder (miconazole)	Y1	L2

Y1   Usually safe when breastfeeding (if applied to nipple and/or areola, clean area with warm water and mild soap before breastfeeding)

Topical Wound and Burn Care Products

Aquaphor Healing Ointment (ceresin/lanolin/mineral oil/petrolatum)	Y1	L2
Bacitracin Ointment (bacitracin)	Y1	L1
Bactine First Aid Liquid/Pain Relieving Cleansing Spray (benzalkonium chloride/lidocaine)	Y2	L3
Betadine Skin Cleanser/Solution (povidone iodine)	N	L4
Boil Ease Ointment (benzocaine/camphor/ichthammol)	Y2	L2
Burn Jel Plus Waterjel (lidocaine)	Y2	L2
Calamine Lotion (calamine/zinc oxide)	Y2	L3
Campho Phenique Gel/Liquid (camphorated phenol)	N	L4
Clorpactin WCS-90 Solution (sodium oxychlorosene)	Y2	L3
Dermoplast Hospital Strength Spray (aloe/lanolin/menthol)	Y2	L1
Double Antibiotic Ointment (bacitracin zinc/polymyxin B sulfate)	Y1	L1
Epsal Drawing Salve Ointment (ichthammol)	Y2	L2
Gold Bond First Aid Quick Spray (benzalkonium chloride/menthol)	Y2	L3
Hibeclens Antiseptic Liquid (chlorhexidine gluconate)	N	L4
Hibistat Hand Antiseptic Wipes (chlorhexidine gluconate/isopropyl alcohol)	N	L4
Hydrogen Peroxide	Y1	L1
Lanacaine Anti-Itch Crème Medication Cream/Maximum Strength Cream Anti-Itch/Maximum Strength First Aid Spray (benzethonium/benzocaine)	Y2	L2
Lidocaine Cream (lidocaine)	Y2	L2
Mederma Cream Plus SPF 30 (octocrylene)	Y1	L2
Mederma Gel (allantoin/allium aloe)	Y2	L2

Neosporin Neo To Go (benzalkonium chloride/pramoxine)	Y2	L3
Neosporin Ointment To Go Ointment (bacitracin/neomycin/polymyxin B)	Y1	L2
Neosporin Plus Pain Relief Cream (neomycin/polymyxin B/pramoxine)	Y2	L2
Neosporin Plus Pain Relief Ointment (bacitracin/neomycin/polymyxin B/pramoxine)	Y2	L2
Newskin Liquid Bandage/Liquid Bandage Spray (8-hydroxyquinolone)	Y2	L2
Newskin Scar Therapy Cream (dimethicone)	Y1	L1
Pedi-Boro Soaks (aluminum sulfate/calcium acetate)	Y2	L1
Petroleum Jelly (white petrolatum)	Y1	L1
Polysporin First Aid Antibiotic Powder/Ointment (bacitracin/polymyxin B)	Y1	L2
Povidone Iodine Ointment/Solution (povidone iodine)	N	L4
PreferOn Stick (allium/dimethicone/urea)	Y1	L2
Prosacea Rosacea Treatment Gel (aloe/sulfur/urea)	Y2	L2
Scarguard MD Liquid (hydrocortisone/silicone/vitamin E)	Y1	L2
Smile's Prid Drawing Salve (ichthammol)	Y2	L2
Solarcaine Cream/Lotion/Spray (benzocaine/triclosan)	Y2	L3
Solarcaine Cool Aloe Burn Relief Gel (aloe/benzocaine)	Y2	L2
Transdermis Scar Therapy Topical Serum (emu oil)	Y1	L2
Triple Antibiotic Ointment (bacitracin/neomycin/polymyxin B)	Yi	L2
Vaseline (white petrolatum)	Y1	L1
Wound Wash Sterile Saline Spray (sodium chloride)	Y1	L1

Y1 *Usually safe when breastfeeding (if applied to nipple and/or areola, clean area with warm water and mild soap before breastfeeding)*

Y2 *Usually safe when breastfeeding (do not apply to breasts)*

N *Avoid when breastfeeding*

Vaginal Products

Clotrimazole 7 Vaginal Cream (clotrimazole)	Y	L1
Gyne-Lotrimin 3 Vaginal Cream (clotrimazole)	Y	L1
Lubrin Vaginal Lubricating Inserts (caprylic-capric triglyceride/glycerin/PEG-6-32/PEG-20/PEG-40/ polysorbate 80)	Y	L2
Massengill Disposable Douche (vinegar/water)	Y	L1
Miconazole 7 Vaginal Cream (miconazole)	Y	L2
Monistat Itch Relief Cream (hydrocortisone)	Y	L2
Monistat 1 Day or Night Combination Pack (miconazole)	Y	L2
Monistat 1 Vaginal Cream (tioconazole)	Y	L2
Monistat 3 Combination Pack (miconazole)	Y	L2
Monistat 3 Vaginal Cream (miconazole)	Y	L2
Monistat 7 Combination Pack (miconazole)	Y	L2
Monistat 7 Vaginal Cream (miconazole)	Y	L2
Replens Vaginal Moisturizer (polycarbophil)	Y	L1
7 Day Vaginal Cream (miconazole)	Y	L2
Summer's Eve Douche (vinegar/water)	Y	L1
Summer's Eve Feminine Cloths (vinegar/water)	Y	L1
Summer's Eve Feminine Wash (citric acid/water)	Y	L1
3 Day Vaginal Cream (clotrimazole)	Y	L1
Tioconazole 1 Day Vaginal Cream (tioconazole)	Y	L2
Vagisil Anti-Itch Cream/Medicated Wipes (aloe/ benzocaine/vitamin A vitamin D/vitamin E)	Y	L2
Vagisil Intimate Moisturizer (aloe/glycerin/chamomile/ propylene glycol)	Y	L2
Vagisil Foaming Wash (mild detergents)	Y	L2
Vagisil Intimate Moisturizer (aloe/glycerin/chamomile/ propylene glycol)	Y	L2
Vagistat 1 Vaginal Cream (tioconazole)	Y	L2

Vagistat 3 Combination Pack (miconazole)	Y	L2
Vagistat 3 Vaginal Cream (miconazole)	Y	L2
Yeast Gard Douche/Feminine Wash/Gel Treatment/Suppositories (probiotics)	Y	L1

Y   Usually safe when breastfeeding

Vitamins and Minerals

Vitamin/Mineral		100% Daily Value	
Vitamin A	Y1	5,000 I.U.	Y1
Beta-Carotene	Y1	3 mg	Y1
Vitamin C	Y1	60 mg	Y1
Vitamin D	Y1	400 I.U.	Y1
Vitamin E	Y1	30 I.U.	Y1
Vitamin K	Y1	80 mcg	Y1
Thiamin (B1)	Y1	1.5 mg	Y1
Riboflavin (B2)	Y1	1.7 mg	Y1
Niacin	Y1	20 mg	Y1
Vitamin B6	Y1	2 mg	Y1
Folic Acid	Y1	400 mcg	Y1
Vitamin B12	Y1	6 mcg	Y1
Biotin	Y1	300 mcg	Y1
Pantothenic Acid	Y1	10 mg	Y1
Calcium	Y1	1000 mg	Y1
Iron	Y1	18 mg	Y1
Phosphorus	Y1	1000 mg	Y1
Iodine	Y1	150 mcg	Y1
Magnesium	Y1	400 mg	Y1
Zinc	Y1	15 mg	Y1
Selenium	Y1	70 mcg	Y1
Copper	Y1	2 mg	Y1
Manganese	Y1	2 mg	Y1
Molybdenum	Y1	75 mcg	Y1
Chromium	Y1	120 mcg	Y1

Y1   *Usually safe when breastfeeding (do not exceed 100% Daily Value)*

Weight Management Products

Product		
AcuTrim Caplets (herbs/minerals/vitamins)	N	L4
Alli Weight Loss Aid Capsules (orlistat)	N	L3
Applied Nutrition Carb Blocker Capsules (caffeine/herbs/white tea extract)	N	L4
Applied Nutrition Green Tea Fat Burner Capsules (chromium/green tea extract/herbs)	N	L4
Applied Nutrition Green Tea Triple Fat Burner Capsules (bioflavanoids/caffeine/herbs/tea extracts/vitamins)	N	L4
Applied Nutrition Natural Fat Burner Capsules (green tea extract/minerals/vitamins)	N	L4
Applied Nutrition 10-Day Hoodia Diet Capsules (amino acids/caffeine/green tea extract/herbs/hoodia)	N	L4
Aqua-Ban Maximum Strength Diuretic Tablets (pamabrom)	Y1	L3
BioLean Accelerator Tablets (herbs/minerals)	N	L4
BioLean Free Tablets (herbs/minerals/vitamins)	N	L4
BioLean II Tablets (caffeine/calcium/herbs)	N	L4
BioMD Nutraceuticals Metabolism T3 Capsules (amino acids/minerals)	N	L4
Biotest Hot-Rox Capsules (amino acids/caffeine/yohimbine)	N	L4
Carb Cutter Original Formula Tablets (ascorbic acid/chromium/green tea extract/herbs)	N	L4
Carb Cutter Phase 2 Starch Neutralizer Tablets (herbs/hydroxycitric acid/vanadium)	N	L4
Dexatrim Max Capsules (caffeine/minerals/tea extracts/vitamins)	N	L4
Dexatrim Max2O Tablets (caffeine/green tea extract/minerals/vitamins)	N	L4
Dexatrim Natural Extra Energy Formula Caplets (caffeine/green tea extract/minerals)	N	L4

Dexatrim Natural Green Tea Formula Caplets (calcium/ chromium/ginseng/green tea extract)	N	L4
Dexatrim Max Complex Capsules (caffeine/chromium/ dehydroepiandrosterone/herbs/tea extracts/vitamins)	N	L4
EAS CLA Capsules (linoleic acid)	Y	L2
Estrin-D Capsules (caffeine/green tea/herbs/magnesium/ vitamin B6)	N	L4
Isatori Lean System 7 Advanced Metabolic Support Formula Capsules (caffeine/green tea/herbs/magnesium/ vitamin B6)	N	L4
Metab-O-Fx Extreme Tablets (herbs/niacin/tea extracts)	N	L4
Metabolife Break Through Tablets (caffeine/cayenne/green tea extract/L-tyrosine)	N	L4
Metabolife Caffeine Free Caplets (garcinia extract/ minerals/ pantothenic acid/vitamins)	N	L4
Metabolife Extreme Energy Capsules (green tea extract/ herbs/magnesium/niacin/pantothenic acid)	N	L4
Metabolife Ultra Caplets (caffeine/co-enzyme Q10/ garcinia extract/minerals)	N	L4
MHP TakeOff Hi-Energy Fat Burner Capsules (green tea extract/herbs)	N	L4
Natrol Carb Intercept with Phase 2 Starch Neutralizer Capsules (white kidney bean extract)	Y	L1
Natrol CitriMax Plus Capsules (calcium/cascara sagrada/ chromium/hydroxycitric acid)	N	L4
Natrol Green Tea 500 mg Capsules (caffeine/catechins/ green tea extract/polyphenols)	N	L4
Natural Balance Fat Magnet Capsules (herbs/lipase/malic acid)	N	L4
Nature Made Chromium Picolinate Extra Strength Tablets (chromium)	N	L4
Nature's Bounty Super Green Tea Diet Capsules (caffeine/ chromium/green tea extract/herbs/vitamin B6)	N	L4
Nature's Bounty Xtreme Lean Zn-Ephedra Free Capsules (amino acids/green tea extract/herbs/ magnesium/ pantothenic acid/vitamins)	N	L4

Nunaturals LevelRight for Blood Sugar Management Capsules (herbs/minerals)	N	L4
One-A-Day Weight Smart Dietary Supplement Tablets (caffeine/green tea/herbs/minerals/pantothenic acid/ vitamins)	N	L4
Prolab Enhanced CLA Tablets (flax seed oil/linoleic acid/ safflower or sunflower oil)	Y	L2
Stacker 2 Ephedra Free Capsules (caffeine/green tea/herbs)	N	L4
Tetrazene ES-50 Ultra High-Energy Weight Loss Catalyst Capsules (amino acids/caffeine/green tea extract/herbs)	N	L4
Tetrazene KGM-90 Rapid Weight Loss Catalyst Capsules (amino acids/olive leaf extract/vitamin B6)	N	L4
Thinz Caplets/Tablets (caffeine/chromium/green tea extract/riboflavin)	N	L4
Twinlab Mega L-Carnitine Tablets (l-carnitine)	N	L3
Twinlab Metabolift Ephedra Free Formula Capsules (amino acids/green tea extract/herbs/minerals/vitamins)	N	L4
Ultra Diet Pep Tablets (green tea extract/herbs/l-tyrosine/ minerals/vitamins)	N	L4
Xtreme Lean Advanced Formula Ephedra Free Capsules (amino acids/caffeine/calcium/flavones/herbs/vitamins)	N	L4
Zantrex 3 Ephedrine Free Tablets (caffeine/herbs/niacin/ rice flour)	N	L4

Y   Usually safe when breastfeeding
Y1   Usually safe when breastfeeding (monitor for decreased milk production; mother should drink extra fluids)
N   Avoid when breastfeeding

Herbals

As with prescription drugs and over the counter (OTC) medications, consumers use herbals to treat a variety of ailments and to maintain health. Herbal use is as prevalent among breastfeeding women as it is with consumers who are not breastfeeding. Herbals provide the opportunity not to use a prescription or OTC medication. In fact, lactation consultants recommend, and breastfeeding mothers take, herbals called galactogogues, to help increase milk supply. Commonly used galactogogues include blessed thistle, chaste tree fruit, fennel, fenugreek, garlic, goat's rue, and milk thistle. Other herbals that may act as galactogogues include alfalfa, anise, borage, caraway, coriander, dandelion, dill, fennel, hops, marshmallow root, nettle, oat straw, red clover, red raspberry, and vervain.

Nursing women who use herbals should approach their use cautiously. The fact that many manufacturers promote their products as "natural" does not always imply that using them is usually safe or compatible with breastfeeding. Unlike the regulation of prescription and OTC medicines, the Food and Drug Administration (FDA) does not regulate herbal products in the same manner. The FDA regulates herbals under food manufacturing regulations. Herbal products are required to be free of contaminants. Herbal labels may not make unfounded health and medical claims. Therefore, there is no government regulation of herbals as drugs, and government-regulated standardization does not exist for herbal preparations.

Because of this situation, active ingredients may be present in more or less amounts than the herbal package label lists. Unknown harmful ingredients may also be present. Strengths of herbal product ingredients may vary depending upon the particular plant used, the part of the plant used, and where, when, and how the herb was processed. These inconsistencies can lead to differences in efficacy and potentially harmful adverse effects in the mother and/or her nursling.

In reality, most knowledge about potential side effects of the wide variety of herbals comes from the systematic collection of data in Germany (e.g., the German Commission E Monographs, which have been translated into English). There have been reports of specific herbal adverse effects, but there is still a lack of standard ways to report these adverse effects. Information provided on the use of herbals should serve as general guidelines for nursing mothers.

As with all medications, breastfeeding women should have a real need for treatment before taking herbal preparations. Depending on the condition being treated, conventional medications should be considered first-line therapy until more controlled studies and data are available for specific herbals.

Herbal Galactogogues

(Used to increase milk supply)

Alfalfa (Medicago sativa) - Y1

Use: Galactogogue, diuretic, laxative
Dose: Up to 60 grams daily (1 to 2 capsules 4 times a day)
Caution: Alfalfa may cause loose stools and/or photosensitivity; do not use if allergic to peanuts and/or legumes; do not use in patients with systemic lupus erythematosus (SLE)

Anise (Anisi fructus) - Y1

Use: Galactogogue, anxiety, antiflatulent
Dose: 3.5 grams to 7 grams as tincture or tea, 5 to 6 times a day
Caution: Anise may cause allergic reaction

Blessed Thistle (Cnici benedicti herba) - Y1

Use: Galactogogue, may increase appetite and settle upset stomach
Dose: Up to 2 grams, in capsule form, daily
Caution: Blessed thistle may cause allergic reaction

Borage (Borago officinalis) - Y1

Use: Galactogogue, anxiety, diuretic
Dose: 1 gram to 2 grams, in capsule form or as tincture, daily
Caution: Borage may cause loose stools and/or minor astrointestinal upset; avoid large amounts due to potential blood thinner action

Caraway (Carvi fructus) - Y

Use: Galactogogue, anxiety, antiflatulent
Dose: 1.5 grams to 6 grams daily as tincture, tea, or essential oil
Caution: Avoid large amounts of the essential oil form

Chaste Tree Fruit, Chasteberry, Vitex (Agni casti fructus) - Y1

Use: Galactogogue, to treat breast pain, for dysmenorrhea
Dose: 30 mg to 40 mg daily as an alcoholic extract (50%-70% alcohol)
Caution: Herb may cause rash; extract form has high alcoholic content, although amount consumed is very small

Coriander, Cilantro (Coriandri fructus) - Y1

Use: Galactogogue, antiflatulent, diuretic, mild antidiabetic
Dose: 3 grams daily as tea
Caution: Herb may rarely cause photosensitivity; avoid herb if allergic to celery; avoid large amounts of herb

Dandelion (Taraxaci herba) - Y1

Use: Galactogogue, antidiabetic, diuretic
Dose: 5 grams, in capsule form or as tincture or tea, 3 times a day
Caution: Dandelion may rarely cause contact dermatitis; patients with bile duct blockage, gall bladder problems, or bowel obstruction should not use

Dill (Anethi fructus) - Y

Use: Galactogogue (aids in milk ejection), antiflatulent, diuretic
Dose: 3 grams daily as tincture or tea
Caution: None

Fennel (Foeniculi fructus) - Y1

Use: Galactogogue, for gastrointestinal disorders, expectorant
Dose: 0.1 mL to 0.6 mL of oil (equal to 100 mg to 600 mg) daily
Caution: Fennel may cause allergic reaction and dermatitis

Fenugreek (Foenugraeci semen) - Y1

Use: Galactogogue, to stimulate appetite, externally to control inflammation
Dose: Orally, 6 grams, in capsule form, daily; externally, 50 grams in 8 ounces of water
Caution: Fenugreek may cause nausea and vomiting in mother and diarrhea in baby; may increase asthma symptoms or lower glucose levels

in mother; may cause skin reactions with external use (avoid nipple area); may cause "maple syrup" smell in mother's and/or baby's urine and/or sweat; do not use if allergic to peanuts and/or legumes

Garlic (Allii sativi bulbus) - Y

Use: Galactogogue, possible positive cardiovascular effects and/or immune system stimulation
Dose: 4 grams to 9 grams, in capsule form, daily
Caution: Garlic may decrease nursing time due to odor in breast milk

Goat's Rue (Galegae officinalis herba) - Y

Use: Galactogogue, lower blood glucose levels
Dose: 1 mL to 2 mL of tincture, 2 to 3 times a day
Caution: None

Hops (Lupuli strobulus) - Y

Use: Galactogogue (aids in milk let down), anxiety, insomnia
Dose: 500 mg of dry extract daily, 1 cup to 2 cups of tea daily, 1 bottle of stout beer daily
Caution: None, but do not use hops if depressed

Marshmallow Root (Althaeae radix) - Y1

Use: Galactogogue, diuretic
Dose: Two (2) 500 mg capsules, in capsule form, 3 times a day; or 60 grams daily as tincture or tea
Caution: Marshmallow root rarely may cause allergic reaction

Milk Thistle (Cardui mariae herba) - Y1

Use: Galactogogue, possible liver protective properties
Dose: 12 grams to 15 grams daily as infusion
(equal to 200 mg to 400 mg of silibinin)
Caution: Milk thistle may have laxative effect and/or cause allergic reaction

Oat Straw, Oats (Avenae stramentum) - Y

Use: Galactogogue, diuretic, anxiety, depression
Dose: 100 grams daily
Caution: Do not use if patient has celiac disease

Red Raspberry (Rubi idaei folium) - Y1

Use: Galactogogue (may increase milk ejection), nutritive
Dose: 2.7 grams as three (3) 300 mg capsules 3 times a day or daily as tincture or tea
Caution: Red raspberry rarely may cause loose stools and/or nausea; may decrease milk supply if used for greater than 2 weeks

Red Clover (Trifolium pretense) - Y

Use: Galactogogue, for estrogenic properties, expectorant
Dose: 40 mg to 80 mg daily as tincture or tea
Caution: Do not exceed recommended dosage; avoid fermented Red Clover; patients taking anticoagulants and/or aspirin should not use (contains coumarin, a blood thinner)

Stinging Nettle (Urtica dioica and Urtica urens) - Y1

Use: Galactogogue, mild diuretic, for mild gastrointestinal upset
Dose: 1.8 grams as one (1) 600 mg capsule 3 times a day, 1 cup of tea 2 to 3 times a day, 2½ mL to 5 mL of tincture 3 times a day
Caution: Stinging nettle may cause mild diuresis and/or mild gastrointestinal upset

Vervain (Verbena officinalis) - Y

Use: Galactogogue, anxiety, hypertension
Dose: 30 grams to 50 grams daily as tea
Caution: Do not use if pregnant due to oxytocic properties

Y   *Usually safe when breastfeeding*
Y1   *Usually safe when breastfeeding (monitor infant for potential side effects)*

Herbals Commonly Used by Women

Aloes (Aloe barbadensis, Aloe ferox, Aloe perryi, Aloe vera) - N

Use: Laxative
Dose: 20 mg to 30 mg daily of hydroxyanthracene (active ingredient) (use lowest effective dose), as powder or water extracts
Caution: Aloes may cause gastrointestinal distress (short term use) and/or electrolyte imbalance, albuminuria, hematuria, potassium deficiency and/or irregular heartbeats; due to side effects, do not use during breastfeeding
Note: Topical gel (Aloe vera) may be safely used for sunburn, minor burns, bug bites, and to soften the skin

Angelica Root, Dong Quai (Angelicae radix) - N

Use: Stimulate the central nervous system, regulation of menstrual cycle (due to antispasmodic and vasodilatation effects)
Dose: 4.5 grams daily, as pulverized herb
Caution: Avoid herb when breastfeeding due to possible phytoestrogenic effect on infant; herb can sensitize skin to light and UV radiation

Bilberry (Vaccinium myrtillus) - N

Use: Eye health
Dose: 60 mg to 160 mg three times a day
Caution: Herb inhibits lactation; do not use during breastfeeding; do not use if taking blood thinners

Buckthorn Bark (Frangulae cortex) and Buckthorn Berry (eR hamni cathartici fructus) - N

Use: Laxative
Dose: 20 mg to 30 mg of hydroxyanthracene (active ingredient)
Caution: Same cautions as for Aloe as a laxative; do not use during breastfeeding

Bugleweed (Lycopi herba) - Y1, Y2

Use: Treat breast pain and/or mild thyroid hyperfunction
Dose: 1 gram to 2 grams (10 mg to 20 mg of extract) daily, as tea
Caution: Herb may decrease prolactin levels; monitor mother and baby for thyroid enlargement after extended exposure

Cascara Sagrada (Rhamni purshianae cortex) - N

Use: Laxative
Dose: 20 mg to 30 mg of hydroxyanthracene (active ingredient)
Caution: Same cautions as for Aloe as a laxative; do not use during breastfeeding

Chamomile Flower (Matricariae flos) - Y

Use: Treat indigestion, as calmative and for relaxation; treat skin and mucous inflammation as a poultice, rinse, or bath additive
Dose: Orally 3 grams, in 5 ounces of boiling water or as 3% to 5% infusion, daily; externally, 50 grams in 1½ gallons of water, as a bath additive, poultice, or rinse
Caution: None

Coltsfoot Leaf (Farfarae folium) - N

Use: Anti-inflammatory during respiratory disturbances
Dose: 4 grams to 6 grams daily (not more than 10 micrograms of pyrrolizidine alkaloids), as pressed juice, tincture, or boiled, strained product
Caution: Do not use during breastfeeding due to possible liver toxicity (do not use for more than 4 to 6 weeks total per year if taken when not breastfeeding)

Comfrey Leaf and Root (Symphytum officinale) - N

Use: Anti-inflammatory agent for bruised areas, sprains, and pulled muscles
Dose: External daily doses should not exceed 100 micrograms of the active ingredient, pyrrolizidine, and its derivatives; used as poultice (extract, pressed juice, crushed roots) or ointment (5% to 20%)
Caution: Avoid if breastfeeding due to liver toxicity and anti-mitotic (affects cell reproduction properties); do not use on sore nipples, breasts, or perineum

Cranberry (Vaccinium macrocarpon) - Y1

Use: Antibacterial and antiseptic to protect against and to resolve urinary tract infections
Dose: 100 mg to 500 mg three times a day
Caution: Generally considered safe when used appropriately; avoid if taking blood thinners

Echinacea Pallida Root (Echinaceae pallidae radix) and Echinacea Purpurea Herb (Echinaceae purpureae herba) - Y

Use: Prevention of common cold, wound healing, treat uncomplicated lower urinary tract infections (UTIs)
Dose: 900 mg, in capsule or tablet form, or as tea or expressed juice, daily
Caution: Usually safe for breastfeeding if used for less than 8 weeks (if used for more than 8 weeks, Echinacea may, in fact, weaken immune-stimulating effects); patients with tuberculosis, HIV, or autoimmune diseases should not use; patients with allergy to sunflowers should not use

Elder Flower (Sambuci flos) - Y

Use: Treat acute upper respiratory infections, diaphoretic (increases sweating), increases bronchial lung secretions
Dose: 10 grams to 15 grams of drug (1 cup to 2 cups of tea) daily, 1.5 grams to 3 grams of fluidextract daily, or 2.5 grams to 7.5 grams of tincture daily
Caution: Elder Flower appears to be safe for breastfeeding as long as only the flowers are used; in sufficient quantities, the seeds are toxic

Ephedra (Ephedrae herba) - N

Use: Vitalizing and stimulating effects, treat asthma and bronchoconstriction, weight loss
Dose: See caution below
Caution: Ephedra can cause vasoconstriction, rapid heart rate, and insomnia, a rapid decrease in effectiveness is possible; addiction is possible; thus, no dose is considered safe Note: FDA ban and court actions have removed Ephedra from market, but illegal or foreign sources may still be available

Evening Primrose Oil (Oenothera biennis) - Y

Use: Anti-inflammatory effects
Dose: 3 grams to 8 grams daily in divided doses (clinical effect may take 8 weeks to 12 weeks)
Caution: Hypersensitivity to herb is possible; herb generally considered to be safe during breastfeeding when used appropriately

Feverfew (Tanacetum parthenium) - N

Use: Treat migraine headaches
Dose: 200 to 300 mg, in capsule or tablet form, daily
Caution: Safety during breastfeeding cannot be assured; mouth sores may occur in 10% of users; taste alterations and lip and tongue swelling and irritation also possible

Flaxseed, Cracked (Not Ground) (Linum usitatissimum) - Y

Use: Laxative
Dose: 1 tablespoonful with 5 ounces of water daily
Caution: May take several days for laxative effects
Note: Flaxseed Oil is a rich source of omega-3 fatty acids, which can prevent skin dryness

Ginger (Zingiber officinale) - Y

Use: Prevent or treat motion sickness, nausea and vomiting, upset stomach
Dose: 2 capsules, as powdered rhizome capsules (500 mg), every 4 hours as needed
Caution: None

Gingko (Ginkgo biloba) - Y1

Use: Treat mental deficiencies of age (decreased memory, decreased concentration, dementia), may enhance learning ability in younger people, may relieve altitude sickness with short-term therapy of 2 days to 3 days pretreatment

Dose: 120 mg, in form of capsules or tablets, in 2 to 3 divided doses daily

Caution: Use with caution when breastfeeding due to potential platelet inhibition, especially with infants with cardiovascular disease and/or mothers already taking a blood thinner; do not use more than 6 weeks to 8 weeks on a one time basis to determine if any benefit exists

Ginseng (Panax ginseng) - N

Use: Enhance mental ability

Dose: 1 gram to 2 grams daily, as cut root or powder, for up to 3 months

Caution: Ginseng may increase blood pressure of breastfeeding mothers who already have hypertension; herb should not be used when breastfeeding due to estrogenic side-effects from ginosenoside components.

Goldenrod (Saldago canadensis, Saldago serotona/ gigantea) - Y

Use: Treat lower urinary tract infections (UTIs)

Dose: 6 grams to 12 grams daily, as botanical preparation or tea

Caution: If used when breastfeeding, drink large amount of water and/or fluids

Grape Seed Extract (Vitis vinifera) - Y

Use: Antioxidant

Dose: Preventative: 50 mg daily; Therapeutic: 150 mg to 300 mg daily

Caution: Hypersensitivity to herb is possible; generally considered to be safe during breastfeeding when used appropriately

Grapefruit Seed Extract (Citrux paradisi) - Y

Use: Treatment of thrush
Dose: 250 mg 3 times a day (liquid extract may also be applied directly to nipples after breastfeeding) (extract has bitter taste)
Caution: Hypersensitivity to herb is possible; generally considered to be safe during breastfeeding when used appropriately

Hawthorn (Crataegus oxyacantha) - N

Use: Hypertension, high cholesterol
Dose: 160 mg to 900 mg in 3 divided doses daily for at least 6 weeks
Caution: No information available for breastfeeding; caution is advised

Indian Snakeroot (Rauwolfiae radix) - N

Use: Treat anxiety, tension, psychomotor irritation, and mild, essential hypertension
Dose: 600 mg daily (contains 6 mg of reserpine), as powder or crushed herb root
Caution: Contraindicated when breastfeeding due to possible central nervous system depression; may cause severe depression due to breakdown of norepinephrine

Kava Kava (Piperis methystici rhizome) - N

Use: Treat nervous anxiety, restlessness
Dose: 60 mg to 120 mg daily, as various herbal forms
Caution: Herb is contraindicated when breastfeeding due to possible central nervous system depression and/or skin discoloration; herb rarely may cause allergic reaction; sedation is possible with large doses; long-term use of very large doses may cause temporary discoloration of skin, hair, and/or nails

Licorice Root (Liquiritiae radix) - N

Use: Treat peptic and duodenal ulcers
Dose: 1.5 grams to 3 grams daily, as liquid or solid dosage forms
Caution: May cause sodium and water retention; may cause low potassium levels; may cause hypertension
Note: These precautions do not apply to eating licorice candy in normal quantities

Passionflower (Passiflorae herba) - Y1

Use: Treat anxiety and insomnia
Dose: 4 grams to 8 grams daily, as tea
Caution: When breastfeeding, monitor infant for possible drowsiness; if infant becomes excessively drowsy, mother should stop taking the herb

Petasites Root (Petasitidis rhizome) - N

Use: Acute spastic urinary tract pain and urinary tract stone pain
Dose: 4.5 grams to 7 grams daily (not more than 1 microgram of pyrrolizidine), as alcohol-based extract
Caution: Herb is contraindicated when breastfeeding due to potential liver toxicity

Psyllium Seed, Blonde (Plantaginis ovatae semen) - Y

Use: Laxative
Dose: 12 grams to 40 grams in 5 ounces of water or juice daily
Caution: Herb may take several days for laxative effects; may disrupt food absorption; may affect insulin dependent patients; may cause allergic reaction

Rhubarb Root (Rhei radix) - N

Use: Laxative
Dose: 20 mg to 30 mg of hydroxyanthracene (active ingredient)
Caution: Same cautions as for Aloe as a laxative; do not use during breastfeeding

Senna Leaf (Sennae folium) and Senna Pod (Sennae fructus) - Y1

Use: Laxative
Dose: 20 mg to 30 mg of hydroxyanthracene (active ingredient)
Caution: Senna safe for breastfeeding as long as it is used on a 1 or 2 times basis, not at a high dose, and not chronically

Siberian Ginseng (Eleutherococcus senticosus) - Y

Use: Enhance mental capacity and combat fatigue
Dose: 2 grams to 3 grams daily, as extract, tea, or Ginseng soda for up to 3 months
Caution: None for breastfeeding; use with caution in mother with hypertension

Soy Lecithin (Lecithinum ex soya) - Y

Use: Treat high cholesterol, treatment of plugged breast ducts
Dose: 3.5 grams, as extract from Fabaceae plant family
Caution: None

St. John's Wort (Hypericum perforatum) - Y1

Use: Orally, to treat depression and anxiety; externally, for wound healing
Dose: Orally, 300 mg (containing 0.3% hypericin) daily, in form of capsules or transdermal patches or as tea; externally, as infusion oil
Caution: When breastfeeding, monitor infant for possible abdominal symptoms (e.g., colic); herb interacts with many drugs

Uva Ursi Leaf, Bearberry (Uvae ursi folium) - N

Use: Urinary tract infections, antimicrobial
Dose: 3 grams (100 mg to 210 mg of hydroquinolone) in 5 ounces of water, as powder for infusions or macerations, up to 4 times daily
Caution: Herb should not be used when breastfeeding due to possible disruption of formation of melanin (if used when not breastfeeding, do not use for more than 7 days due to decreased formation of melanin)

Valerian Root (Valerianae radix) - Y1

Use: Anxiety, as a sleep aid
Dose: 2 grams to 3 grams, in form of capsules or as a tea, taken in divided doses daily
Caution: When breastfeeding, monitor infant for possible drowsiness; if infant becomes excessively drowsy, mother should stop taking the herb

Y   *Usually safe when breastfeeding*
Y1   *Usually safe when breastfeeding (monitor infant for potential side effects)*
Y2   *Usually safe when breastfeeding (may decrease prolactin level)*
N   *Avoid when breastfeeding*

Herbs Contraindicated in Breastfeeding Mothers and Their Recommended Alternatives

Herb	Typical Use	Recommended Alternative
	Major Galactogogues	Blessed Thistle*, Chaste Tree Fruit*, Fennel*, Fenugreek*, Garlic, Goat's Rue, Milk Thistle*
	Minor Galactogogues	Alfalfa*, Anise*, Borage*, Caraway, Coriander*, Dandelion*, Dill, Fennel*, Hops, Marshmallow Root*, Oat Straw, Red Clover, Red Raspberry*, Stinging Nettle*, Vervain
Comfrey	Analgesics	Bugleweed*,**
Feverfew	Anti-Inflammatory/ Headache (Migraine) Agents	Evening Primrose Oil*
Coltsfoot	Cough, Cold, and Allergy Products	Echinacea, Elder Flower
Ephedra	Anti-Asthmatic Preparations	
Aloes, Buckthorn, Cascara Sagrada, Licorice, Rhubarb	Gastrointestinal Agents	Chamomile, Flaxseed, Psyllium Seed (Blonde), Senna*

	Nausea and Vomiting Preparations	Ginger
Hawthorn	Lipid Lowering Agents	Soy Lecithin
Bearberry, Petasites, Uva Ursi	Urinary Tract Infection Preparations	Cranberry*, Goldenrod
	Thrush Agents	Grapefruit Seed*
Indian Snakeroot, Kava Kava	Anti-Anxiety Agents	Passionflower*, St. John's Wort*, Valerian*
Angelica Root, Dong Quai, Ginseng Root	Stimulants	Ginkgo Biloba*, Siberian Ginseng
	Sleep Aid Preparations	Melatonin
	Antioxidants	Grape Seed*
Bilberry	Eye Health Products	

*- Monitor nursling for potential side effects
**- May decrease prolactin level

Common Dietary Supplements

Alpha Lipoic Acid - N

Use: Coenzyme with antioxidant and antidiabetic properties
Dose: 600 mg daily in two or three divided doses; maintenance, 200 mg to 600 mg daily in single or divided doses
Caution: Coenzyme not recommended for use during breastfeeding

Bromelain - Y1

Use: Proteolytic enzymes used for anti-inflammatory, antitumor, and digestive properties
Dose: 500 mg to 2,000 mg daily in divided doses
Caution: Scientific studies for safety during breastfeeding are not available; very large molecular size should greatly limit passage into breast milk; pediatric doses exist; hypersensitivity possible; enzyme may increase heart rate at higher doses

Chondroitin Sulfate - Y

Use: Protective effects on cartilage
Dose: 800 mg to 1,200 mg daily in single or divided doses
Caution: No pediatric concerns reported via breast milk; very large molecular size should greatly limit passage into breast milk

Coenzyme Q - Y1

Use: Antioxidant and cardiotonic
Dose: 150 mg to 600 mg daily in divided doses
Use: No pediatric concerns reported via breast milk; large molecular size should limit passage into breast milk; pediatric doses exist; hypersensitivity possible; avoid high doses

Glucosamine - Y1

Use: Osteoarthritis
Dose: 1,500 mg daily in single or divided doses
Caution: No pediatric concerns reported via breast milk; supplement has low oral bioavailability; maternal plasma levels are almost undetectable; observe for gastrointestinal disturbances

Glutamine - Y1

Use: Metabolic fuel, digestive disorders
Dose: 7 grams to 30 grams daily in divided doses
Caution: Scientific studies for safety during breastfeeding are not available; very large molecular size and maternal protein metabolism should limit passage into breast milk; pediatric doses exist; observe for gastrointestinal disturbances

Immunizen Powder Capsules (arabinogalactan/colostrum/lactoferrin/yeast/beta-glucans) - Y

Use: Boosts immune system
Dose: 6 capsules with water 1 to 2 hours before meals for 10 days as needed
Caution: Product may cause gastrointestinal discomfort

Lutein - N

Use: Antioxidant, for eye health, macular degeneration prevention
Dose: 10 mg daily
Caution: No human data available for contraindications, precautions, drug interactions, or adverse reactions

Lysine - Y

Use: Recurrent herpes simplex infections
Dose: 1 gram to 2 grams daily in divided doses
Caution: No pediatric concerns reported via breast milk; maternal supplementation should not result in significant levels in breast milk; pediatric doses exist

Melatonin - Y

Use: Treat insomnia, to prevent jet lag
Dose: 1 mg to 10 mg daily, in various oral forms of 0.5 mg to 5 mg, including extended release formulations
Caution: No pediatric concerns reported via breast milk; mothers with autoimmune disorders, diabetes, and/or depression should avoid use; breastfeeding mothers should not take more than 3 mg daily

Omega-3 Fatty Acids - Y

Use: Cardiovascular benefits
Dose: Limit of 2 grams daily from dietary supplements
Caution: Safe at normal doses for maternal use during breastfeeding

Probiotics - Y

Use: Diarrhea, gastrointestinal colonization, urinary tract infections, vaginal candidiasis, bacterial vaginosis
Dose: Depends upon use (see label)
Caution: Observe for gastrointestinal disturbances; probiotic potential of lactobacilli, isolated from milk of healthy mothers, is similar to that of the strains commonly used in commercial probiotic products; pediatric doses exist

Quercetin - N

Use: Antioxidant
Dose: 2 grams every two hours for a maximum of two days (acute allergic symptoms) or 2 grams daily (chronic allergies)
Caution: Neurotoxicity is dose-limiting adverse effect; observe for hypersensitivity

SAMe - N

Use: Depression, pain disorders, liver conditions
Dose: 200 mg to 1,600 mg daily
Caution: No data available for use while breastfeeding; more breastfeeding compatible preparations are available for these conditions

Y   *Usually safe when breastfeeding*
Y1   *Usually safe when breastfeeding (monitor infant for potential side effects)*
N   *Avoid when breastfeeding*

Breastfeeding and Medications Websites

American Academy of Pediatrics Policy Statement: The Transfer of Drugs and Other Chemicals Into Human Milk: http://aappolicy. aappublications.org/cgi/reprint/pediatrics;108/3/776.pdf

The AAP policy statement provides important concepts regarding the use of cigarettes, psychotropic drugs, and silicone implants while a mother is breastfeeding. It is well referenced, and seven tables regarding the statement are provided.

Breastfeeding Online: www.Breastfeedingonloine.com

Cindy Curtis, a Registered Nurse and International Board Certified Lactation Consultant (IBCLC) developed the website to help empower women to choose to breastfeed and to educate society of the importance and benefits of breastfeeding. She provides therapies for mastitis, thrush, engorgement, insufficient milk supply, and nipple vasospasm among others.

LactMed Search: toxnet.nlm.nih.gov/cgi-bin/sis/htmlgen?LACT

Philip O. Anderson, a leading pharmacist breastfeeding expert, originated LactMed as a peer-reviewed and fully referenced National Library of Medicine database of drugs to which breastfeeding mothers may be exposed. Maternal and infant levels of drugs, possible effects on breastfed infants and on lactation, and alternate drugs to consider can be found on this website.

MICROMEDEX Healthcare Series: http://www.micromedex.com/ products/hcs/

For most drugs in MICROMEDEX, current information and corresponding references are listed under the category, "Breast Feeding". If insufficient information is listed under this category, it can be found under the category, "Pharmacokinetics" with the subsections, "Distribution", "Metabolism", and "Excretion".

Natural Standards: http://www.naturalstandard.com/

http://www.naturalstandard.com/naturalstandard/monographs/
herbssupplements/
For pertinence to breastfeeding and lactation, the herbs and supplement monographs all have a pregnancy and lactation section. However, safety data often suggest that it is not safe since data is not available.

http://www.naturalstandard.com/naturalstandard/monographs/
alternativemodalities/
Another section of the website provides monographs to specific therapies and practices. This section does not, however, have information pertaining to breastfeeding and lactation.

http://www.naturalstandard.com/naturalstandard/monographs/
conditions/
When clicking on the "Effectiveness" button on the top of the website, it takes you to a list of practices, diseases, and conditions. This section of the website specifically covers topics such as breastfeeding, breast milk stimulants (or lactation stimulation), and breast reduction. The topics do not have monographs, but do provide a list of related practices organized by validity according to scientific evidence.

Natural Medicines Comprehensive Database (NMCD) Overview:
www.naturaldatabase.com

This website contains a large selection of natural medicines, each with a detailed monograph. The monographs provide the common names, scientific names, uses, safety details, adverse reactions, interactions with drugs, food, other herbs and supplements, diseases/conditions, and dosage of the particular medicine. Within the safety section of the monograph, a pregnancy and lactation section provides how "likely" the medication is to be safe to consume while pregnant or lactating, even though data is often not available. The likelihood of safety in lactation is often backed up with the general uses or the amount contained in a normal diet.

Nice Breastfeeding: www.nicebreastfeeding.com

The Nice Breastfeeding website provides counseling tips for pharmacists (included in this book), as well as a compilation of useful breastfeeding websites. Healthcare professionals may contact Dr. Nice for consultation advice at no cost through the website.

Infant Risk Center: www.infantrisk.org

Dr. Hale is currently considered a leading expert in the use of medications in breastfeeding women. Dr. Hale offers answers to questions by healthcare professionals only, through a medication forum on his website. However, the information is accessible by the public. In addition to the medication forum, a wealth of breastfeeding information is compiled.

Index

Symbols

3 Day Vaginal Cream 93
4-Way Fast Acting Nasal
    Decongestant Spray 58
4-Way Mentholated Nasal
    Decongestant Spray 58
4-Way Saline Moisturizing Mist 58
7 Day Vaginal Cream 93
454 Maximum Strength Gel 21

A

Abreva Cold Sore 67
Abreva Fever Blister Treatment 67
Abreva Pump Cold Sore 67
Absorbine Jr. Back Patch 21
Absorbine Jr. Liniment 21
Acetaminophen Tablets 23
Acetic Acid Otic Solution 70
Acne 19
Actidose-Aqua Suspension 23
Actidose with Sorbitol Suspension 23
Actifed Cold & Allergy Tablets 35
Activated Charcoal 27
ActivOn Ultra Strength Backache
    Roll-On Liquid 21
Act Mouthwash 67
AcuTrim Caplets 96
Advanced Solutions Acne Mark
    Fading Peel with CelluZyme 19
Advil 23
Advil Allergy Sinus Caplets 35
Advil Cold & Sinus Caplets 35
Advil Cold & Sinus Liqui-Gels 35
Afrin No Drip All Night 12 Hour
    Pump Mist 58
Afrin No Drip Extra Moisturizing
    Nasal Spray 58
Afrin No Drip Original Pump Mist
    Nasal Spray 58

Afrin No Drip Severe Congestion
    Nasal Spray 58
Afrin No Drip Sinus Nasal Spray 58
Agni casti fructus 102
Aim Toothpaste 67
Akurza 34
Alavert 24-Hour Allergy Tablets 35
Alavert D-12 Hour Allergy and Sinus
    Tablets 35
Alavert Oral Disintegrating Tablets
    35
Alcohol 17
Alconefrin Nasal Drops 58
Aleve 23
Aleve-D Cold & Sinus Caplets 35
Aleve Sinus & Headache Caplets 35
Alfalfa 101, 113
Alka-Seltzer Effervescent Antacid and
    Pain Reliever 23
Alka-Seltzer Morning Relief Tablets
    23
Alka-Seltzer Plus Cold & Cough
    Liquid 35
Alka-Seltzer Plus Cold & Cough
    Liquid Gels 35
Alka-Seltzer Plus Cold Original
    Effervescent Tablets 35
Alka-Seltzer Plus Day Cold Liquid
    Gels 35
Alka-Seltzer Plus Day & Night Cold
    Formula Effervescent Tablets 35
Alka-Seltzer Plus Day & Night Liquid
    Gels 35
Alka-Seltzer Plus Flu Effervescent
    Tablets 35
Alka-Seltzer Plus Mucus &
    Congestion Effervescent Tablets 36
Alka-Seltzer Plus Night Cold Formula
    Effervescent Tablets 35
Alka-Seltzer Plus Night Cold Formula
    Liquid Gels 35

Alka-Seltzer Plus Night Cold Liquid 35
Alka-Seltzer Plus Sinus Formula Effervescent Tablets 36
Allerest Maximum Strength Tablets 36
Allerest No Drowsiness Allergy & Sinus Caplets 36
Allerest PE Allergy & Sinus Relief Tablets 36
Allergy 35
Allergy Buster Nasal Spray 58
Allii sativi bulbus 103
Alli Weight Loss Aid Capsules 96
Aloe barbadensis 105
Aloe ferox 105
Aloe perryi 105
Aloes 105
Aloe vera 105
Alophyn Enteric Coated Stimulant Laxative Pills 55
Alpha Keri Cream 73
Alpha Keri Original Lotion 73
Alpha Keri Shower & Bath Oil 73
Althaeae radix 103
Americaine Hemorrhoidal Ointment 52
Aminobenzoic acid (PABA) 84
Amlactin Moisturizing Cream 73
Amlactin Moisturizing Lotion 73
Amlactin XL Moisturizing Lotion 73
Ammonium Lactate Lotion 73
Amosan Oral Wound Cleanser Powder Packs 67
Anacin 81 Tablets 51
Anacin Advanced Headache Tablets 23
Anacin Aspirin Free Extra Strength Tablets 23
Anacin Fast Pain Relief Maximum Strength Tablets 23
Anacin Fast Pain Relief Tablets 23
Analgesic Balms 21
Analgesics 23
Anbesol Cold Sore Therapy Ointment 67
Anbesol Gel 67
Anbesol Liquid 67
Anbesol Maximum Strength Gel 67

Anbesol Maximum Strength Liquid 67
Anbesol Regular Strength Gel 67
Anbesol Regular Strength Liquid 67
Anethi fructus 102
Angelicae radix 105
Angelica Root 105
Anise 101, 113
Anisi fructus 101
Antacid 27
Antidiarrheal 31
Antiflatulant 27
Anti-Plaque Dental Rinse 67
Antipyretics 23
Anusol HC Ointment 52
Anusol Suppositories 52
Applied Nutrition 10-Day Hoodia Diet Capsules 96
Applied Nutrition Carb Blocker Capsules 96
Applied Nutrition Green Tea Fat Burner Capsules 96
Applied Nutrition Green Tea Triple Fat Burner Capsules 96
Applied Nutrition Natural Fat Burner Capsules 96
Aqua-Ban Maximum Strength Diuretic Tablets 96
Aqua Care Lotion 73
Aquafresh Sensitive Toothpaste 67
Aquafresh Toothpaste 67
Aquafresh White Trays 67
Aquaphor Healing Ointment 73, 91
Aquaphor Original Ointment 73
Arm & Hammer Toothpaste 67
ArthriCare Cream 21
Arthritis Hot Crème 21
Arthritis Pain Relief Caplets 23
Artificial Sweeteners 5, 32
Ascriptin Maximum Strength Tablets 23
Ascriptin Regular Strength Tablets 23
Aspen 83
Aspercin Tablets 23
Aspercreme Cream 21
Aspercreme Lotion 21
Aspirin 325 mg Tablets 23
Aspirin 500 mg Tablets 23
Aspirin Free Pain Relief Tablets 23

Aspirin Tablets 51
Asthma 33
Asthmahaler Mist Inhaler 33
Asthma Mist Inhaler 33
Asthmanephrin 33
Auralgan Ear Drops 70
Auro-Dri Ear Drying Aid 70
Auro Ear Drops 70
Aveeno Anti-Itch Concentrated
    Lotion 86
Aveeno Bath Treatment 73
Aveeno Calamine & Pramoxine HCl
    Anti-Itch Cream 86
Aveeno Clear Complexion Bar 19
Aveeno Creamy Moisturizing Oil 73
Aveeno Daily Moisturizer Ultra-
    Calming APF 15 73
Aveeno Daily Moisturizing Lotion 73
Aveeno Hydrocortisone 1% Anti-Itch
    Cream 86
Aveeno Intense Relief Hand Cream
    73
Aveeno Intense Relief Overnight
    Cream 73
Aveeno Moisturizing Bar for Dry
    Skin 73
Aveeno Moisturizing Lotion Skin
    Relief 73
Aveeno Positively Radiant
    Moisturizing Lotion 73
Aveeno Positively Radiant
    Moisturizing Lotion SPF 15 73
Aveeno Positively Smooth
    Moisturizing Lotion 73
Aveeno Radiant Skin Daily
    Moisturizer with SPF 15 73
Aveeno Skin Relief Body Wash
    Fragrant Free 73
Aveeno Skin Relief Moisturizing
    Cream 74, 86
Aveeno Ultra-Calming Night Cream
    74
Avenae stramentum 103
Avobenzone 84
Axsain Cream 21
Ayr Allergy & Sinus Nasal Mist 58
Ayr Saline Nasal Gel No-Drip Sinus
    Spray 58

Ayr Saline Nasal Gel With Soothing
    Aloe 58
Ayr Saline Nasal Mist 58

B

Bacitracin Ointment 91
Back-Quell Tablets 23
Back Ultra Strength Patch 21
Bactine First Aid Liquid 91
Bactine Original First Aid Liquid 86
Bactine Pain Relieving Cleansing
    Spray 86, 91
Balneol Hygienic Cleansing Lotion
    52
Bayer Back & Body Pain Caplets 23
Bayer Extra Strength Caplets 24
Bayer Extra Strength Plus Caplets 24
Bayer Genuine Tablets 24
Bayer Low Dose Aspirin Chewable
    Tablets 51
Bayer Low Dose Aspirin Safety
    Coated Tablets 51
Bayer Safety Coated Caplets 24
Bayer Women's Low Dose Aspirin
    Caplets 51
BC Arthritis Strength Powders 24
BC Original Strenth Powders 24
Bearberry 112
Benadryl Allergy Kapgels 36
Benadryl Allergy Quick Dissolve
    Strips 36
Benadryl Allergy & Sinus Headache
    Kapgels 36
Benadryl Allergy & Sinus Kapgels 36
Benadryl Allergy Ultratabs 36
Benadryl Capsules 61
Benadryl-D Allergy & Sinus Tablets
    36
Benadryl Extra Strength Itch Stopping
    Cream 86
Benadryl Extra Strength Itch Stopping
    Relief Stick 86
Benadryl Extra Strength Spray 86
Benadryl Gel 86
Benadryl Itch Stopping Extra Strength
    Gel 86
Benadryl Liquid 61
Benadryl Liqui-Gels 36

Benadryl Original Strength Itch
  Stopping Cream 86
Benadryl Severe Allergy & Sinus
  Headache Caplets 36
Benadryl Tablets 61
Benefiber Plus Calcium Powder 55
Benefiber Powder 55
Benefiber Stick Packs Powder 55
Bengay Arthritis Cream 21
Bengay Cream 21
Benylin Adult Formula Cough Syrup
  36
Benylin All-In-One Cold & Flu
  Nighttime Syrup 36
Benylin All-In-One Cold & Flu
  Syrup 36
Benylin Chest Coughs Non-Drowsy
  Cough Syrup 36
Benylin Cold & Sinus Plus Caplets
  36
Benylin Cold & Sinus Rapid-Gels 36
Benylin Cold & Sinus Tablets 36
Benylin DM-D-E Chest Cough &
  Cold Syrup 37
Benylin DM Dry Cough Syrup 36
Benylin DM-E Chest Cough & Cold
  Syrup 37
Benylin DM-E Chest Cough Syrup
  37
Benylin E Chest Congestion Syrup
  37
Benylin Extra Strength Cough &
  Cold Syrup 37
Benzedrex Inhaler 46
Benzodent Cream 67
Benzophenone-9 84
Benzoyl Peroxide Bar 19
Beta-Carotene 95
Betadine Skin Cleanser 91
Betadine Solution 91
Big Red 83
Bilberry 105
BioLean Accelerator Tablets 96
BioLean Free Tablets 96
BioLean II Tablets 96
BioMD Nutraceuticals Metabolism
  T3 Capsules 96
Biore Blemish Fighting Ice Cleanser
  19

Biotest Hot-Rox Capsules 96
Biotin 95
Bisacodyl Tablets 55
Blessed Thistle 101, 113
Body Clear Body Scrub 19
Boil Ease Ointment 91
Bonine Chewable Tablets 61
Borage 101, 113
Borago officinalis 101
Bromo-Seltzer Powders 24
Bronkaid Caplets 33
Bronkaid Mist Inhaler 33
Bronkotabs 33
Buckley's Cough Mixture 37
Buckthorn Bark 105
Buckthorn Berry 105
Bufen Tablets 24
Bufferin Extra Strength Tablets 24
Bufferin Tablets 24
Bugleweed 106, 113
Burn Jel Plus Waterjel 91

C

Caffeine 17, 83
Caladryl Anti-Itch Lotion 86
Caladryl Clear Anti-Itch Lotion 86
CalaGel Anti-Itch Gel 86
Calamine Lotion 86, 91
Calcium 95
Callus 34
Calmol 4 Hemorrhoidal Suppositories
  52
Calm-X Tablets 61
Campho-Phenique Cold Sore Gel 67
Campho Phenique Gel 91
Campho Phenique Liquid 91
Canada Dry Diet Cola 83
Canada Dry Jamaica Cola 83
Capzasin-HP Crème 21
Caraway 101, 113
Carb Cutter Original Formula Tablets
  96
Carb Cutter Phase 2 Starch
  Neutralizer Tablets 96
Cardui mariae herba 103
Carmol-10 Cream 74
Carmol-10 Lotion 74
Carters Laxative Sodium Free Pills 55

Carvi fructus 101
Cascara Sagrada 106
Cascara Sagrada Tablets 55
Castor Oil 55
Celestial Seasonings Soothers Herbal
Throat Drops 46
Ceo-Two Evacuant Suppositories 55
Cepacol Sore Throat Lozenges 46
Cepacol Sore Throat Spray 46
Cepastat Sore Throat Lozenges 46
Cetaphil Daily Advance Ultra
Hydrating Lotion 74
Cetaphil Daily Facial Moisturizer SPF
15 with Parsol 1789 74
Cetaphil Moisturizing Cream 74
Cetaphil Moisturizing Lotion 74
Cetaphil Therapeutic Hand Cream
74
Cetaphil UVA-UVB Defense SPF
50 74
Chamomile 113
Chamomile Flower 106
Chasteberry 102
Chaste Tree Fruit 102, 113
Cheracol-D Syrup 37
Cheracol Sore Throat Spray 46
Chill Factor Cleansing Pads 20
Chloraseptic Pocket Pump Sore
Throat Spray 67
Chloraseptic Sore Throat Lozenges
46
Chloraseptic Sore Throat Spray 46
Chlor-Trimeton 4-Hour Allergy
Tablets/Redi-Tabs 37
Chromium 95
Cilantro 102
Cinoxate 84
Citrucel Caplets 52, 55
Citrucel Powder 52, 55
Citrux paradisi 110
Claritin 24 Hour Allergy &
Congestion Tablets 37
Claritin 24 Hour Allergy Tablets 37
Claritin-D 12 Hour Allergy &
Congestion Tablets 37
Clean & Clear Advantage Acne Spot
Treatment 19
Clean & Clear Blackhead Cleansing
Scrub 19
Clean & Clear Blackhead Clearing
Daily Cleansing Pads 19
Clean & Clear Continuous Control
Acne Cleanser 19
Clearasil Acne Treatment Tinted
Cream 19
Clearasil Stay Clear Acne Fighting
Cleansing Wipes 19
Clearasil Stay Clear Daily Facial Scrub
19
Clearasil Stay Clear Daily Pore
Cleansing Pads 19
Clearasil Stay Clear Skin Perfecting
Wash 19
Clearasil Stay Clear Stay Clear Oil-
Free Gel Wash 19
Clearasil Stay Clear Vanishing Acne
Treatment Cream 19
Clearasil Ultra Acne Clearing Gel
Wash 19
Clearasil Ultra Acne Clearing Scrub
19
Clearasil Ultra Acne Rapid Action
Treatment Vanishing Cream 19
Clear Complexion Foaming Cleanser
19
Clearly Confident Triple Action
Fungus Treatment Cream 89
Clear Pore Oil-Eliminating Astringent
19
Clorpactin WCS-90 Solution 91
Close-Up Mouthwash 67
Close-Up Toothpaste 67
Clotrimazole 7 Vaginal Cream 93
Clotrimazole Cream 89
CM Plex Cream 21
Cnici benedicti herba 101
Coca-Cola 83
Cocoa Butter Stick 74
Coffee 82
Coke 83
Colace Capsules 52, 55
Colace Glycerin Suppositories for
Adults and Children 55
Colace Liquid 52, 55
Colace Syrup 52, 55
Cold 35
Colgate Simply White Gel 67
Colgate Toothpaste 67

127

Coltsfoot Leaf 106
Comfrey Leaf 106
Comfrey Root 106
Commit Stop Smoking 2 mg
  Lozenges 81
Commit Stop Smoking 4 mg
  Lozenges 81
Common Dietary Supplements 115
Compound W 34
Comtrex Day & Night Severe Cold &
  Sinus Caplets 37
Comtrex Deep Chest Cold Caplets
  37
Comtrex Non-Drowsy Cold &
  Cough Caplets 37
Contac Cold & Flu Non-Drowsy
  Maximum Strength Caplets 37
Contact Cold & Flu Day & Night
  Caplets 37
Contact Cold & Flu Maximum
  Strength Caplets 37
Continuous Control Acne Wash Oil-
  Free 19
Copper 95
Coriander 102, 113
Coriandri fructus 102
Coricidin HBP Chest Congestion &
  Cough Softgels 37
Coricidin HBP Cold & Flu Tablets
  38
Coricidin HBP Cough & Cold
  Tablets 37
Coricidin HBP Maximum Strength
  Flu Tablets 38
Coricidin HPB Day-Night Multi-
  Symptom Tablets 38
Coricidin HPB Nighttime Multi-
  Symptom Cold Relief Liquid 38
Corn 34
Corn Huskers Lotion 74
Correctol Tablets 55
Cortaid Advanced 12-Hour Anti-Itch
  Cream 86
Cortaid Intensive Therapy Cooling
  Spray 86
Cortaid Maximum Strength Cream
  86
Cortaid Maximum Strength
  Ointment 86

Cortaid ntensive Therapy
  Moisturizing Cream 86
Cortaid Poison Ivy Care Toxin
  Removal Cloths 86
Cortaid Poison Ivy Care Treatment
  Kit 86
Corticool Gel 86
Cortizone-10 Cool Relief Gel 87
Cortizone-10 Creme 87
Cortizone-10 Creme Plus 87
Cortizone-10 Easy Relief Applicator
  87
Cortizone-10 Intensive Healing
  Formula 87
Cortizone-10 Maximum Strength
  Anti-Itch Ointment 87
Cortizone-10 Ointment 87
Cough and Cold Inhalers 46
Cranberry 107, 114
Crataegus oxyacantha 110
Crest Sensitivity Toothpaste 67
Crest Toothpaste 67
Crest Whitestrips 68
Cruex Cream 89
Cruex Powder 89
Cruex Prescription Strength Cream
  89
Cruex Prescription Strength Lotion
  89
Cruex Prescription Strength Powder
  89
Cruex Prescription Strength Spray 89
Cruex Spray 89
Curel Continuous Comfort Fragrance
  Free Lotion 74
Curel Continuous Comfort Original
  Formula Lotion 74
Curel Natural Healing Nourishing
  Lotion 74
Curel Natural Healing Soothing
  Lotion 74
Curel Ultra Healing Intensive
  Moisture Lotion 74

D

Daily Facials Lathering Cleansing Cloths-Clarifying for Combination-Oily Skin 20
DairyEnz Capsules 28
DairyGest Lactozymes Capsules 28
Dandelion 102, 113
Dandrex Shampoo 48
Dandruff 48
Datril Tablets 24
DDS-Acidophilus Capsules 28
Debrox Ear Drops 70
Delsym 12 Hour Cough Relief Liquid 38
Denorex Dandruff Daily Protection Shampoo 48
Denorex Dandruff Extra Strength Shampoo 48
Denorex Therapeutic Protection 2-in-1 Shampoo 48
Denorex Therapeutic Protection Shampoo 48
Dermarest Eczema Medicated Lotion 87
Dermarest Psoriasis Medicated Moisturizer 48
Dermarest Psoriasis Medicated Overnight Treatment 48
Dermarest Psoriasis Medicated Shampoo-Conditioner 48
Dermarest Psoriasis Medicated Skin Treatment 48
Dermarest Psoriasis Scalp Treatment 48
Dermoplast Hospital Strength Spray 91
Desenex Antifungal Liquid Spray 89
Desenex Antifungal Powder 89
Desenex Antifungal Spray 89
Desenex Cream 89
DeWitt's Pills Tablets 24
Dexatrim Max2O Tablets 96
Dexatrim Max Capsules 96
Dexatrim Max Complex Capsules 97
Dexatrim Natural Extra Energy Formula Caplets 96
Dexatrim Natural Green Tea Formula Caplets 97

DHS SAL Shampoo 48
DHS Tar Dermatological Hair & Scalp Shampoo 48
DHS Tar Gel Shampoo 48
DHS Tar Shampoo 48
DHS Zinc Shampoo 48
Diar Aid Caplets 31
Diar Aid Tablets 31
Diarrest Tablets 31
Diasorb Capsules 31
Diasorb Tablets 31
Diatrol Tablets 31
Dicarbosil Tablets 28
Diet Coke 83
Diet Pepsi 83
Diet Rite 83
Di-Gel Tablets 28
Digestive Aid 27
Dill 102, 113
Dimetapp Cough & Cold Long-Acting Liquid 38
Dimetapp Elixir Cold & Allergy 38
Dimetapp Nighttime Cold & Congestion Liquid 38
Dioxybenzone 84
Doan's Extra Strength Caplets 24
Docusol Constipation Relief Mini Enemas 52, 55
Domeboro Astringent Solution Powder Packets 87
Dong Quai 105
Donnagel Suspension 31
Double Antibiotic Ointment 91
Doxidan Tablets 55
Dramamine Chewable Tablets 61
Dramamine Less Drowsy Formula Tablets 61
Dramamine Original Tablets 61
Dristan 12 Hour Nasal Spray 58
Dristan Cold Multi-Symptom Tablets 38
Dristan Nasal Spray 58
Drixoral 12 Hour Cold & Allergy Tablets 38
Dr Pepper 83
Dr. Scholl's Callus Remover 34
Dr. Scholl's Clear Away Wart Remover 34

Dr. Scholl's Corn and Callus Remover 34
Dr. Scholl's Corn Remover 34
Dr. Scholl's Freeze Away 34
Dr. Snapz Swabplus Mouth Sore Relief Swabs 68
Drug Labeling 15
Dulcolax Stool Softener Capsules 52, 55
Dulcolax Suppositories/Tablets 55
Duofilm 34
Duoplant Corn Remover 34
Durasal Solution 34
Duration 12 Hour Spray 58
Dynafed IB Tablets 24
Dynafed IB Tablets EX 24
Dyspel Tablets 24

E

Ear Medications 70
EAS CLA Capsules 97
Ecamsule 84
Echinacea 113
Echinaceae pallidae radix 107
Echinaceae purpureae herba 107
Echinacea Pallida Root 107
Echinacea Purpurea Herb 107
Ecotrin Low Strength Tablets 51
Ecotrin Regular Strength Tablets 24
Efidac 24 Capsules 38
Efidac 24 Chlorpheniramine Tablets 38
Efidac 24 (R) Capsules 38
Elder Flower 107, 113
Eleutherococcus senticosus 111
Emagrin Tablets 24
Emetrol Cherry Syrup 61
Empirin Tablets 24
ENTSOL Buffered Hypertonic Nasal Irrigation Mist 58
ENTSOL Buffered Hypertonic Saline Nasal Spray 58
ENTSOL Nasal Gel with Aloe and Vitamin E 58
Ephedra 107
Ephedrae herba 107
Epsal Drawing Salve Ointment 91
Epsom Salts 55

Equal 32
Equalactin Chewable Tablets 31, 52, 55
e Rhamni cathartici fructus 105
Estrin-D Capsules 97
Eucerin Cream Original 74
Eucerin Dry Skin Therapy Calming Cream 74
Eucerin Lotion Daily Replenishing 74
Eucerin Lotion Original 74
Eucerin Plus Intensive Repair Hand Cream 74
Eucerin Plus Intensive Repair Lotion 74
Eucerin Plus Smoothing Essentials 74
Eucerin Redness Relief Daily Perfecting Lotion SPF 15 75
Eucerin Redness Relief Soothing Cleanser 75
Eucerin Redness Relief Soothing Moisture Lotion SPF 15 75
Eucerin Redness Relief Soothing Night Cream 75
Eucerin Sensitive Facial Skin Gentle Hydrating Cleanser 75
Evac-Q-Kwik Bowel Cleansing System 55
Evening Primrose Oil 108, 113
Excedrin Back & Body Capsules 24
Excedrin Extra Strength Caplets 24
Excedrin Extra Strength Express Gels 24
Excedrin Extra Strength Geltabs 24
Excedrin Extra Strength Tablets 24
Excedrin Migraine Caplets 24
Excedrin Migraine Geltabs 24
Excedrin Migraine Tablets 24
Excedrin Sinus Headache Caplets 38
Excedrin Tension Headache Caplets 24
Excedrin Tension Headache Express Gels 24
Excedrin Tension Headache Geltabs 24
Ex-Lax Maximum Strength Tablets/ Tablets 55
Ex-Lax Ultra Stimulant Laxative Tablets 55

Eye Medicines 62
EZ-Char Pellets 24

F

Facewipes to Go with Acne
   Medication 20
Facial Bar 5% 20
Farfarae folium 106
Fennel 102, 113
Fenugreek 102, 113
Feverall Adult Strength Suppository
   24
Feverfew 108
Fiberall Powder 55
Fibercon Caplets 31, 52
Fibercon Tablets 55
Flaxseed 113
Flaxseed, Cracked 108
Fleet Bisacodyl Enema 55
Fleet Enema 56
Fleet Enema Extra 56
Fleet Mineral Oil Enema 56
Fleet Sof-Lax Softgels 56
Fleet Sof-Lax Tablets 52
Fleet Stimulant Laxative Tablets 56
Fleet Suppositories 55
Flexall 454 Gel 21
Flexall Plus Maximum Strength Gel
   21
Flu 35
Fluorigard Rinse 68
Foeniculi fructus 102
Foenugraeci semen 102
Folic Acid 95
Frangulae cortex 105
Freezone Wart Treatment 34
FungiCure Anti-Fungal Gel 89
FungiCure Anti-Fungal Liquid 89
FungiCure Intensive Spray 89
FungiCure Manicure-Pedicure
   Formula Liquid 89
FungiCure Maximum Strength Anti-
   Fungal Liquid Spray 89
FungiCure Professional Formula
   Liquid 89
Fungi Nail Anti-Fungal Solution 89

G

Galegae officinalis herba 103
Garlic 103, 113
GasAid Maximum Strength Anti-Gas
   Softgels 28
Gas-X Antigas Chewable Tablets 28
Gas-X Antigas Softgels 28
Gas-X Antigas Thin Strips 28
Gas-X Extra Strength with Maalox
   Chewable Tablets 28
Gaviscon Regular Extra Strength
   Tablets 28
Gaviscon Regular Strength Liquid 28
Gaviscon Regular Strength Tablets 28
G.B.H. Shampoo 71
Gelusil Chewable Tablets 28
Ginger 108, 114
Gingko 109
Ginkgo biloba 109
Ginkgo Biloba 114
Ginseng 109
Glutamine 116
Glycerin Suppositories 56
Gly-Oxide Liquid 68
Goat's Rue 103, 113
Gold Bond Extra Strength Medicated
   Body Lotion 87
Gold Bond First Aid Quick Spray 91
Gold Bond Medicated Body Lotion
   87
Gold Bond Medicated Extra Strength
   Powder 87
Gold Bond Medicated Maximum
   Strength Anti-Itch Cream 87
Gold Bond Medicated Powder 87
Gold Bond Quick Spray 87
Gold Bond Ultimate Comfort Body
   Powder 75
Gold Bond Ultimate Healing Lotion
   75
Goldenrod 109, 114
Goody's Body Pain Formula Powders
   24
Goody's Extra Cool Orange Powders
   25
Goody's Extra Strength Headache
   Powders 25
Gordochom Solution 89

Gordofilm Wart Remover Solution
34
Grapefruit Seed 114
Grapefruit Seed Extract 110
Grape Seed 114
Grape Seed Extract 109
Guaifed Capsules 39
Guaitab Tablets 39
Gyne-Lotrimin 3 Vaginal Cream 93

H

Habitrol Nicotine Transdermal
System Patch Step 1 81
Habitrol Nicotine Transdermal
System Patch Step 2 81
Habitrol Nicotine Transdermal
System Patch Step 3 81
Halfprin 81 mg Tablets 51
Halfprin 162 mg Tablets 51
Halls Cough Drops 46
Haltran Tablets 25
Hawthorn 110
Headache and Migraine Products 23
Head & Shoulders Citrus Breeze
Dandruff Conditioner 48
Head & Shoulders Citrus Breeze
Dandruff Shampoo 48
Head & Shoulders Citrus Breeze
Dandruff Shampoo Plus
Conditioner 48
Head & Shoulders Classic Clean
Dandruff Conditioner 48
Head & Shoulders Classic Clean
Dandruff Shampoo 48
Head & Shoulders Classic Clean
Dandruff Shampoo Plus
Conditioner 48
Head & Shoulders Dandruff Intensive
Treatment Shampoo 48
Head & Shoulders Dry Scalp Care
Dandruff Conditioner 48
Head & Shoulders Dry Scalp Care
Dandruff Shampoo 48
Head & Shoulders Dry Scalp
Care Dandruff Shampoo Plus
Conditioner 48
Head & Shoulders Extra Volume
Dandruff Shampoo 48

Head & Shoulders Intensive
Treatment Shampoo 49
Head & Shoulders Ocean Lift
Dandruff Shampoo 49
Head & Shoulders Ocean Lift
Shampoo Plus Dandruff
Conditioner 49
Head & Shoulders Refresh Dandruff
Shampoo 49
Head & Shoulders Refresh Dandruff
Shampoo Plus Conditioner 49
Head & Shoulders Restoring Shine
Dandruff Shampoo 49
Head & Shoulders Restoring
Shine Dandruff Shampoo Plus
Conditioner 49
Head & Shoulders Sensitive Care
Dandruff Shampoo 49
Head & Shoulders Sensitive
Care Dandruff Shampoo Plus
Conditioner 49
Head & Shoulders Smooth & Silky
Dandruff Conditioner 49
Head & Shoulders Smooth & Silky
Dandruff Shampoo 49
Head & Shoulders Smooth &
Silky Dandruff Shampoo Plus
Conditioner 49
Healthprin Adult Low Strength
Aspirin Tablets 51
Healthprin Full Strength Tablets 25
Healthprin Half Dose Aspirin Tablets
51
Heart Attack 51
Heartburn 27
Hemorrhoidal Preparations 52
Hemspray Hemorrhoidal Relief Spray
52
Herbal Galactogogues 101
Herbals 99
Herb-Lax Tablets 56
Herpecin-L Lip Balm Stick 68
Hibeclens Antiseptic Liquid 91
Hibistat Hand Antiseptic Wipes 91
HOLD Lozenges 46
Homosalate 84
Hops 103, 113
Humbid Capsules 39

Humbid DM Sustained-Release
Capsules 39
Humbid E Oral Tablets 39
Humbid LA Capsules 39
Humco Cola Syrup 61
Hydrisalic Gel 34
Hydrocil Instant Fiber Laxative
Powder 56
Hydrocortisone Cream 0.5%/1% 87
Hydrocortisone Lotion 1% 87
Hydrocortisone Ointment 0.5%/1%
87
Hydrogen Peroxide 91
Hydrogen Peroxide Rinse 68
Hyland's Cough Syrup 39
Hyland's C-Plus Cold Tablets 39
Hyland's Diarrex Tablets 31
Hyland's Earache Drops 70
Hyland's Leg Cramps with Quinine
Caplets 25
Hyland's Leg Cramps with Quinine
Sublingual Tablets 25
Hyland's Restful Legs Tablets 25
Hypericum perforatum 112

I

Ibuprofen 200 mg Tablets 25
Ibuprohm Max Tablets 25
Ibuprom Max Tablets 25
Ice Roll-On 21
Icy Hot 21
Immunizen Powder Capsules 116
Imodium A -D Caplets 31
Imodium A -D E-Z Chews 31
Imodium A -D Liquid 31
Imodium Multi-Symptom Relief
Caplets 31
Imodium Multi-Symptom Relief
Chewable Tablets 31
Indian Snakeroot 110
Infrarub Ointment 21
Innerclean Herbal Blend 56
Innerclean Herbal Tablets 56
Insulin 54
Insulin Preparations 5
Intal Inhaler 58
Iodine 95
Ionil Plus Conditioning Shampoo 49

Ionil-T Plus Shampoo 49
Ionil-T Shampoo 49
Iron 95
Isatori Lean System 7 Advanced
Metabolic Support Formula
Capsules 97
Isopentenyl-4-methoxycinnamate 84
Ivarest Double Relief Formula 87
Ivy Block Lotion 87
Ivy-Dry Anti-Itch Cream with Zytrel
87
Ivy-Dry Cream with Zytrel 87
Ivy-Dry Scrub with Zytrel 87
Ivy-Dry Super with Zytrel 87

J

Johnson's Baby Oil 75
Johnson's Baby Powder 75
JointFlex Cream 21
Jolt 83

K

Kank-A Mouth Pain Liquid 68
Kank-A Soft Brush Tooth Mouth Pain
Gel 68
Kank-A Soothing Beads 68
Kao-Paverin Capsules 31
Kaopectate Advanced Formula
Suspension 31
Kaopectate Extra Strength Liquid 31
Kaopectate Liquid 31
Kaopectate Liqui-Gels 52, 56
Kaopectate Maximum Strength
Tablets 31
Kaopectate Tablets 31
Kaopek Suspension 31
Kava Kava 110
Kellogg's Castor Oil 56
Keralyt Gel 34
Keri Age Defy & Protect Lotion 75
Keri Long Lasting Hand Cream 75
Keri Lotion Sensitive Skin 75
Keri Moisture Therapy Advance Extra
Dry Skin Lotion 75
Keri Nourishing Shea Butter Lotion
75
Keri Original Formula Lotion 75

133

Keri Overnight Deep Conditioning Lotion 75
Keri Renewal Milk Body Lotion 75
Keri Renewal Serum for Dry Skin 75
Ketoconazole Cream 89
Kewll Shampoo 71
Kick 83
Kondremul Emulsion 56
Konsyl-D Powder 52, 56
Konsyl Easy Mix Powder 52, 56
Konsyl Fiber Caplets 31, 56
Konsyl Orange Powder 52, 56
Konsyl Original Powder 52, 56
Konsyl Senna Prompt Capsules 56
K-Pek Suspension 31

L

Lac-Hydrin Five Lotion 75
Lactaid Fast Act Capsules 28
Lactaid Fast Act Chewable Tablets 28
Lactaid Original Tablets 28
Lactase Capsules 28
Lactinex Granules 28
Lactinex Tablets 28
Lamasil AT Continuous Spray 89
Lamasil AT Cream 89
Lamasil AT Gel 89
Lanacaine Antibacterial First Aid Spray 87
Lanacaine Anti-Itch Crème Medication Cream 91
Lanacaine Anti-Itch Ultra Moisturizing Maximum Strength Cream 87
Lanacaine Maximum Strength Cream 87
Lanacaine Maximum Strength Cream Anti-Itch 91
Lanacaine Maximum Strength First Aid Spray 91
Lanacaine Original Strength Cream 87
Lanolin Ointment Hydrous 75
Laxatives 55
Lecithinum ex soya 112
Lice Freee! Gel 71
LiceMD Liquid 71
Lice Shield Spray Shampoo 71

Licorice Root 110
Lidocaine Cream 91
Lindane Lotion 71
Lindane Shampoo 71
Linum usitatissimum 108
Liquid Lactase Drops 28
Liquiritiae radix 110
Long Acting Cough Thin Strips 43
L'Oreal Homme Purete Anti-Dandruff Shampoo 49
Lotrimin AF Antifungal Aerosol Liquid Spray 89
Lotrimin AF Antifungal Athlete's Foot Cream 89
Lotrimin AF Antifungal Jock Itch Aerosol 89
Lotrimin AF Antifungal Powder 89
Lotrimin AF For Her Antifungal Cream 89
Lotrimin Ultra Antifungal Cream 89
Lozenges 46
Lubricant Eye Drops 65
Lubriderm Advanced Therapy Hand Cream 76
Lubriderm Advanced Therapy Moisturizing Lotion 76
Lubriderm Advanced Therapy Triple Smoothing Lotion 76
Lubriderm Daily Moisture Fragrance Free Lotion 76
Lubriderm Daily Moisture Lotion 76
Lubriderm Daily Moisturizer Lotion SPF 15 76
Lubriderm Intense Skin Repair Body Cream 76
Lubriderm Intense Skin Repair Body Lotion 76
Lubriderm Intense Skin Repair Body Lotion with Itch Relief 76
Lubriderm Sensitive Skin Therapy Moisturizing Lotion 76
Lubriderm Skin Nourishing Moisturizing Lotion with Premium Oat Extract 76
Lubriderm Skin Nourishing Moisturizing Lotion with Sea Kelp Extract 76

Lubriderm Skin Nourishing Moisturizing Lotion with Shea and Cocoa Butter 76
Lubrin Vaginal Lubricating Inserts 93
Lupuli strobulus 103
Lutein 116
Lycopi herba 106
Lysine 116

M

Maalox Advanced Maximum Strength Chewable Tablets 28
Maalox Advanced Maximum Strength Liquid 28
Maalox Advanced Regular Strength Liquid 28
Maalox Regular Strength Chewable Tablets 28
Maalox Total Relief Liquid 31
Maalox Total Relief Maximum Strength Relief Liquid 28
Mack's Dry-n-Clear Ear Drying Aid 70
Magnesium 95
Magnesium Citrate Solution 56
Magsal Tablets 25
Maltsupex Liquid 56
Manganese 95
Marezine For Motion Sickness Tablets 61
Marshmallow Root 103, 113
Massengill Disposable Douche 93
Matricariae flos 106
Mederma Cream Plus SPF 30 91
Mederma Gel 91
Medicago sativa 101
Melatonin 114, 116
Mello Yello 83
Mentadent Toothpaste 68
Metab-O-Fx Extreme Tablets 97
Metabolife Break Through Tablets 97
Metabolife Caffeine Free Caplets 97
Metabolife Extreme Energy Capsules 97
Metabolife Ultra Caplets 97
Metamucil Capsules 52
Metamucil Original Texture Powder 52

Metamucil Original Texture Powder-Orange 56
Metamucil Smooth Texture Powder-Orange 52, 56
Metamucil Wafers 52, 56
Methyl anthranilate 84
Methylbenzylidene camphor 84
Mexoryl XL 84
MG217 Medicated Lotion 49
MG217 Ointment 49
MG217 Tar Shampoo 49
MHP TakeOff Hi-Energy Fat Burner Capsules 97
Micatin Cream 89
Miconazole 7 Vaginal Cream 93
Miconazole Cream 89
Midol IB Cramp Relief Formula Tablets 25
Midol Menstrual Complete Caplets 25
Midol Menstrual Complete Gelcaps 25
Midol Teen Formula Caplets 25
Milk Thistle 103, 113
Mineral Ice Gel 21
Mineral Oil 76
Minerals 95
Miracle of Aloe Miracure Anti-Fungal Liquid 89
Mobigesic Tablets 25
Molybdenum 95
Monistat 1 Day or Night Combination Pack 93
Monistat 1 Vaginal Cream 93
Monistat 3 Combination Pack 93
Monistat 3 Vaginal Cream 93
Monistat 7 Combination Pack 93
Monistat 7 Vaginal Cream 93
Monistat Itch Relief Cream 93
Mosco Callus & Corn Remover Liquid 34
Motion Sickness 61
Motrin IB Caplets 25
Motrin IB Sinus Tablets 39
Motrin IB Tablets 25
Mountain Dew 83
Mouthwashes 69
Mr Pibb 83

Mucinex Cold Mixed Berry Liquid 39

Mucinex Cough Orange Crème Mini-Melts 39

Mucinex D Extended-Release Tablets 39

Mucinex DM Extended Release Tablets 39

Mucinex Full Force Nasal Spray 58

Mucinex Maximum Strength Tablets 39

Murine Ear Wax Removal System 70

Muro 128 Ointment 64

Muro 128 Solution 64

Mylanta Gas Maximum Strength Chewable Tablets 28

Mylanta Maximum Strength Liquid 28

Mylanta Regular Strength Liquid 28

Mylanta Supreme Antacid Liquid 29

Mylanta Ultimate Strength Chewable Tablets 29

Mylanta Ultimate Strength Liquid 29

Myoflex Cream 21

N

Naphazoline Plus Eye Drops 64

Naphcon-A Eye Drops 64

Naphcon Eye Drops 64

Nasal Comfort 58

NasalCrom Nasal Allergy Symptom Prevention and Controller Nasal Spray 58

Nasal Moist Nasal Gel 58

Nasal Moist Nasal Spray 58

Nasal Preparations 58

Natrol Carb Intercept with Phase 2 Starch Neutralizer Capsules 97

Natrol CitriMax Plus Capsules 97

Natrol Green Tea 500 mg Capsules 97

Natural Balance Fat Magnet Capsules 97

Nature Made Chromium Picolinate Extra Strength Tablets 97

Nature's Bounty Super Green Tea Diet Capsules 97

Nature's Bounty Xtreme Lean Zn-Ephedra Free Capsules 97

Nature's Tears 64

Nausea 61

Nauzene Chewable Tablets 61

Neo Heliopan AP 84

Neosporin AF Athlete's Foot Antifungal Spray Liquid 89

Neosporin AF Athlete's Foot Antifungal Spray Powder 89

Neosporin AF Athlete's Foot Cream 89

Neosporin AF Jock Itch Antifungal Cream 89

Neosporin Neo To Go 92

Neosporin Ointment To Go Ointment 92

Neosporin Plus Pain Relief Cream 92

Neosporin Plus Pain Relief Ointment 92

Neo-Synephrine Extra Strength Nasal Spray 59

Neo-Synephrine Mild Formula Nasal Spray 59

Neo-Synephrine Nighttime Nasal Spray 59

Neotame 32

Nephrox Suspension 29

Neutrogena Acne Stress Control 3-in-1 Hydrating Acne Treatment 19

Neutrogena Blackhead Eliminating Daily Scrub 19

Neutrogena Blackhead Eliminating Foaming Pads 19

Neutrogena Clear Pore Cleanser Mask 19

Neutrogena Deep Moisture Body Cream 76

Neutrogena Norwegian Formula Body Moisturizer 76

Neutrogena Norwegian Formula Deep Moisture Hand Cream 76

Neutrogena Norwegian Formula Hand Cream 76

Neutrogena Original Formula Shampoo 49

Neutrogena Scalp Build-Up Control Shampoo 49

Neutrogena Stubborn Itch Control Shampoo 49
Neutrogena T-Gel Daily Control 2-in-1 Dandruff Shampoo Plus Conditioner 49
Neutrogena T-Gel Daily Control Dandruff Shampoo 49
Neutrogena T-Gel Extra Strength Shampoo 49
Neutrogena Triple Clean Anti-Blemish Astringent 19
Neutrogena Triple Clean Anti-Blemish Pads 19
Neutrogena T/Sal Therapeutic Conditioner 49
Newskin Liquid Bandage 92
Newskin Liquid Bandage Spray 92
Newskin Scar Therapy Cream 92
Niacin 95
Nica Patches 81
N'ICE Lozenges 46
Nicoderm CQ Step 1 Clear Patch 81
Nicoderm CQ Step 2 Clear Patch 81
Nicoderm CQ Step 3 Clear Patch 81
Nicorelief Gum 81
Nicorette 2 mg Patch 81
Nicorette 4 mg Patch 81
Nicorette Gum 81
Nicorette Lozenges 81
Nicorette Mini Lozenges 81
Nicorrete Plus Gum 81
Nicotine 18
Nicotine Gum 81
Nicotine Lozenges 81
Nicotine Transdermal System Patches 81
Nicotrol Gum 81
Nicotrol Patches 81
Nivea Body Age Defying Formula Deep Moisturizer For Body 76
Nivea Body Original Moisture Daily Lotion Dry Skin 77
Nivea Cream 77
Nivea Essentially Enriched Lotion 77
Nivea Smooth Sensation Body Oil 77
Nivea Smooth Sensation Daily Lotion Dry Skin 77
Nix Cream Rinse 71
Nizoral Anti-Dandruff Shampoo 49

Nizoral Cream 90
No Doz Tablets 82
Nose Better Natural Mist Moisturizing Spray 59
Nose Better Non-Greasy Aromatic Relief Gel 59
Nostrilla Complete Congestion Relief Nasal Spray 59
Nostrilla Conditioning Double Moisture Nasal Spray 59
Nostrilla Original Fast Relief Nasal Spray 59
Novahistine DMX Elixir 39
Novahistine Elixir 39
Novitra Cold Sore Maximum Strength Cream 68
Noxzema Triple Clean Anti-Bacterial Lathering Cleanser 20
Nunaturals LevelRight for Blood Sugar Management Capsules 98
Nupercainal Cream 52
Nupercainal Ointment 52
Nuprin Cream 21
Nuprin Tablets 25
NutraSweet 32

O

Oats 103
Oat Straw 103, 113
Occlusal-HP 34
Ocean Premium Saline Nasal Spray 59
Octocrylene 84
Octyl methoxycinnamate 84
Octyl salicylate 84
Ocucoat Eye Drops 64
Ocucoat PF Eye Drops 64
Oculotect Eye Drops 64
Ocu-Tears 64
Oenothera biennis 108
Oil Free Acne Stress Control Power Clear Scrub 19
Oil Free Acne Wash Cleansing Cloths 19
Oil Free Acne Wash Cream Cleanser 19
Oil Free Acne Wash Foam Cleanser 19

Oil Free Anti-Acne Moisturizer 19
Olay Body Wash 20
Olay Maximum Daily Cleansing
   Pads 20
Olay Maximum Face Scrub 20
Olay Regenerist Daily Regenerating
   Cleanser 20
Omega-3 Fatty Acids 117
One-A-Day Weight Smart Dietary
   Supplement Tablets 98
On-the-Spot Acne Treatment
   Vanishing Formula 19
Opcon-A Allergy Relief Drops 64
Opcon-A Eye Drops 64
Ophthalmics 62
Opti-Clear Eyewash 64
Opti-Clear Redness Reliever Eye
   Drops 64
Opticrom Allergy Eye Drops 64
Optics Laboratory Minidrops Eye
   Therapy 64
Orabase with Benzocaine Gel 68
Orabase with Benzocaine Paste 68
Orajel Antiseptic Mouth Sore Rinse
   68
Orajel Medicated Mouth Cold Sore
   Brush 68
Orajel Medicated Mouth Sore Swabs
   68
Orajel Mouth Sore Medicine Gel 68
Orajel Protective Mouth Sore Discs
   68
Orajel Ultra Mouth Sore Medicine
   Film-Forming Gel 68
Oral Balance Gel 68
Oral Balance Liquid 68
Oral Hygiene 67
Orudis KT Capsules 25
Oscillococcinum Pellets 39
Otics 70
Otrivin Nasal Drops 59
Otrivin Nasal Spray 59
Oxybenzone 84
Oxy Chill Factor Daily Wash 20
Oxy Chill Maximum Daily Wash 20
Oxy Chill Spot Treatment 20

P

Padimate O 84
Pain Relief Patch 21
Pamprin All Day Caplets 25
Pamprin Cramp Caplets 25
Pamprin Max Caplets 25
Pamprin Multi-Symptom Caplets 25
Panadol Extra Tablets 25
Panadol Tablets 25
Panax ginseng 109
PanOxyl Aqua Gel Maximum
   Strength Gel 20
PanOxyl Bar 10% Maximum
   Strength 20
Panscol 34
Pantene Pro-V Anti-Dandruff
   Shampoo + Conditioner 49
Pantothenic Acid 95
Parepectolin Suspension 31
Parsol SLX 84
Passiflorae herba 111
Passionflower 111, 114
Pedi-Boro Soaks 92
Pediculosis (Lice) Treatments 71
Pepcid AC Gelcaps 29
Pepcid AC Maximum Strength Chews
   29
Pepcid AC Maximum Strength
   Tablets 29
Pepcid AC Tablets 29
Pepcid Complete Chewable Tablets
   29
Pepsi-Cola 83
Pepsi Light 83
Pepsodent Powder 68
Pepsodent Toothpaste 68
Pepto Bismol Caplets 31, 61
Pepto-Bismol Caplets 29
Pepto-Bismol Cherry Maximum
   Strength Liquid 29
Pepto Bismol Chewable Tablets 31,
   61
Pepto-Bismol Instacool Peppermint
   Chewable Tablets 29
Pepto Bismol Liquid 61
Pepto BismolLiquid 31
Pepto Bismol Liquid Max 31, 61

Pepto-Bismol Maximum Strength
Liquid 29
Pepto-Bismol Original Chewable
Tablets 29
Pepto-Bismol Original Liquid 29
Percogesic Extra Strength Caplets 25
Percogesic Original Strength Caplets
25
Perdiem Overnight Relief Tablets 56
Peri-Colace Tablets 56
Permethrin Lotion 71
Peroxyl Rinse 68
Persia-Gel 10 Maximum Strength 19
Pert 2-in-1 Dandruff Dismissed
Shampoo 50
Pert Plus Dandruff Control Shampoo
Plus Conditioner 50
Pertussin DM Extra Strength Cough
Syrup 39
Petasites Root 111
Petasitidis rhizome 111
Peterson's Ointment 52
Petroleum Jelly 77, 92
Phazyme 95 Capsules 29
Phazyme 95 Tablets 29
Phenylbenzimidazole sulfonic acid 84
Phillips Antacid 56
Phillips Cramp-Free Laxative Caplets
56
Phillips Laxative Chewable Tablets 56
Phillips Milk of Magnesia
Concentrated Liquid 56
Phillips Milk of Magnesia Liquid 56
Phillips Milk of Magnesia Suspension
29
Phillips Milk of Magnesia Tablets 29
Phillips M-O Liquid 56
Phillips Stool Softener Capsules 52,
56
Phisoderm Anti-Blemish Body Wash
20
pHisoderm Cream Cleanser 77
Phos Flur Rinse 68
Phosphorus 95
Physicians' Choice Ear Wax Removal
Kit 70
Pibb Xtra 83
Pinworm Treatments 72

Pin-X Pinworm Treatment Suspension
72
Piperis methystici rhizome 110
Plantaginis ovatae semen 111
Plax Rinse 68
Polysporin First Aid Antibiotic
Ointment 92
Polysporin First Aid Antibiotic
Powder 92
Pond's Cold Cream 77
Pore Treatment Gel 20
Povidone Iodine Ointment 92
Povidone Iodine Solution 92
PreferOn Stick 92
Premsyn PMS Caplets 26
Preparation H Anti-Itch Cream 52
Preparation H Hemorrhoidal Cooling
Gel 52
Preparation H Hemorrhoidal Cream
Maximum Strength Pain Relief 52
Preparation H Hemorrhoidal
Ointment 53
Preparation H Hemorrhoidal
Suppositories 53
Preparation H Medicated Wipes 53
Pretz Moisturizing Nasal Spray 59
Prilosec OTC Tablets 29
Primatene Mist Inhaler 33
Primatene Tablets 33
Privine Nasal Spray 59
Probiotics 117
Procto Foam-HC Spray 53
Procto Foam Spray 53
Prodium Tablets 26
ProFar Ear Drops 70
Prolab Enhanced CLA Tablets 98
Pronto Plus Pinworm Treatment
Suspension 72
Prosacea Rosacea Treatment Gel 92
pseudoephedrine 41
P&S Liquid/Shampoo 49
Psoriasin Gel 50
Psoriasin Liquid Dab-On 50
Psoriasin Ointment 50
Psoriasin Therapeutic Shampoo and
Body Wash 50
Psoriasis 48
Psyllium Seed 113
Psyllium Seed, Blonde 111

139

Q

Quercetin 117

R

Rapid Clear Acne Defense Face Lotion 19
Rauwolfiae radix 110
RC Cola 83
Re-Azo Tablets 26
Rectacaine Hemorrhoidal Ointment 53
Red Clover 104
Red Raspberry 104, 113
Reese's Pinworm Treatment Suspension 72
Reese's Pinworm Treatment Tablets 72
Refenesen Chest Congestion & Pain Relief Caplets 40
Refenesen Chest Congestion & Pain Relief PE Caplets 40
Refenesen Chest Congestion Relief Caplets 40
Refresh Celluvisc 64
Refresh Classic 64
Refresh Eye Itch Relief 64
Refresh Lacri-Lube 64
Refresh Liquigel 64
Refresh Optive/Optive Sensitive 64
Refresh Plus 64
Refresh P.M. 64
Refresh Tears 64
Regu-Lax Drops 56
Regu-Lax Forte Tablets 56
Regu-Lax Tablets 57
Releev 1-Day Cold Sore Treatment 68
Relief Eye Drops 64
Rembrandt Canker Sore Toothpaste 69
Rembrandt Toothpaste 69
Rembrandt Whitening Gel 69
Rembrandt Whitening Strips 69
Replens Vaginal Moisturizer 93
Respitrol Liquid 33
Rhamni purshianae cortex 106
Rheaban Tablets 31

Rhei radix 111
Rhubarb Root 111
Riboflavin (B2) 95
RID Lotion 71
RID Spray 71
Rincinol P.R.N. Rinse 69
Riopan Plus Suspension 29
Riopan Plus Suspension Plus Tablets 29
Rite Aid Lice Pyrinyl Shampoo 71
Robitussin Chest Congestion Liquid 40
Robitussin Cough & Chest Congestion DM Liquid 40
Robitussin Cough & Chest Congestion DM Max Liquid 40
Robitussin Cough & Chest Congestion Sugar-Free DM Liquid 40
Robitussin Cough & Cold CF Liquid 40
Robitussin Cough & Cold D Liquid 40
Robitussin Cough & Cold Long-Acting Liquid 40
Robitussin Cough Drops 46
Robitussin CoughGels Liqui-Gels 40
Robitussin Cough Long-Acting Liquid 40
Robitussin Night Time Cough, Cold & Flu Liquid 40
Robitussin Night Time Cough & Cold Liquid 40
Robitussin Sugar Free Throat Drops 46
Rohto V Arctic Eye Drops 64
Rohto V Cool Redness Relief Drops 64
Rohto V Ice Eye Drops 64
Rohto Zi For Eyes Lubricant Eye Drops 64
Rolaids Antacid & Antigas Soft Chews 29
Rolaids Extra Strength Plus Gas Soft Chews 29
Rolaids Extra Strength Soft Chews 29
Rolaids Extra Strength Tablets 29
Rolaids Multi-Symptom Chewable Tablets 29

Rolaids Tablets 29
Rubi idaei folium 104

S

SalAcid Plasters 34
Salactic Film 34
Saldago canadensis 109
Saldago serotona/gigantea 109
Salicylic Acid Film 34
Salicylic Gel 34
Salicylic Liquid 34
Salicylic Solution 34
Salinex Nasal Lubricant 59
Salinex Nasal Spray 59
Salonpass Arthritis Pain Patch 21
Sal-Plant Gel 34
Sambuci flos 107
SAMe 117
Sarna Sensitive Lotion 87
Sarna Ultra Anti-Itch Cream 87
Scalpicin Anti-Itch Liquid Scalp
    Treatment 50
Scalpicin Maximum Strength Liquid
    50
Scarguard MD Liquid 92
Scot-Tussin Diabetes CF Sugar-Free
    Liquid 40
Scot-Tussin DM 40
Scot-Tussin DM Maximum Strength
    Sugar-Free Liquid 40
Scot-Tussin Original Sugar-Free
    Liquid 40
Scot-Tussin Senior Sugar-Free Liquid
    40
Sebex Shampoo 50
Seborrhea 48
Sebulex Medicated Dandruff
    Shampoo 50
Selenium 95
Selsun Blue 2-in-1 Dandruff
    Shampoo 50
Selsun Blue Dandruff Shampoo 50
Selsun Blue Dandruff Shampoo Plus
    Conditioner 50
Selsun Blue Medicated Treatment
    Dandruff Shampoo 50
Selsun Blue Moisturizing Formula
    Dandruff Shampoo 50

Selsun Blue Naturals Dandruff
    Shampoo 50
Selsun Blue Normal to Oily Formula
    Dandruff Shampoo 50
Selsun Salon 2-in-1 Pyrithione Zinc
    Shampoo 50
Selsun Salon Shampoo Plus
    Conditioner 50
Senna 113
Sennae folium 111
Sennae fructus 111
Senna Leaf 111
Senna Pod 111
Senokot S Tablets 57
Senokot Tablets 57
Senokot XTRA Tablets 57
Sensitive Skin Pads Alcohol Free 20
Sensodyne Toothpaste 69
Serutan Granules 57
Shasta Cherry Cola 83
Shasta Cola 83
Shasta Diet Cherry Cola 83
Shasta Diet Cola 83
Siberian Ginseng 111, 114
Silphen Cough Syrup, Old Formula
    41
Similasan Dry Eye Relief Eye Drops
    65
Similasan Ear Wax Relief Ear Drops
    70
Similasan Hay Fever Relief Non-
    Drowsy Formula Nasal Spray 59
Similasan Pink Eye Relief Eye Drops
    65
Similasan Stye Eye Relief Eye Drops
    65
Simply Cough Liquid 41
Simply Saline Sterile Saline Nasal
    Mist 59
Simply Stuffy Liquid 41
Sinarest Drops 41
Sinarest Nasal Spray 59
Sinarest Syrup 41
Sinarest Tablets 41
Sine-Aid IB Tablets 41
Sine-Aid Maximum Strength Tablets
    41
Sine-Off Multi Symptom Relief Cold
    Cough Medicine Tablets 41

Sine-Off Multi Symptom Relief Severe Cold Medicine Tablets 41
Sine-Off Non-Drowsy Relief Maximum Strength Caplets 41
Sine-Off Strong, Fast Relief Sinus Cold Medicine Caplets 41
SinoFresh Nasal & Sinus Care Spray 59
Sinus Buster Nasal Spray 59
Sinutab Sinus Caplets 41
Skin Lubricants and Moisturizers 73
Sleep Aid Preparations 79
Smile's Prid Drawing Salve 92
Smoking Cessation Aids 81
Social Drug Overview 17
Soda 83
Sodium Bicarbonate Powder 29
Sodium Bicarbonate Tablets 29
Soft Drink 83
Solarcaine Aloe Extra Burn Relief Gel 87
Solarcaine Aloe Extra Burn Relief Spray 87
Solarcaine Cool Aloe Burn Relief Gel 92
Solarcaine Cream 92
Solarcaine First Aid Medicated Spray 88
Solarcaine Lotion 92
Solarcaine Spray 92
Soothe Lubricant Eye Drops 65
Soothe XP Emollient Lubricant Eye Drops 65
Soy Lecithin 112, 114
Splenda 32
Sportscreme Cream 21
Stacker 2 Ephedra Free Capsules 98
Stanback Headache Powders 26
Steri-Optics Eyewash 65
Stevia In The Raw 32
Stimulants 82
Stinging Nettle 104, 113
St. Ives Medicated Apricot Scrub 20
St. John's Wort 112, 114
St. Joseph Chewable Aspirin Tablets 51
St. Joseph Enteric Safety-Coated Tablets 51
Stool Softeners 55

Stridex Essential Pads with Salicylic Acid 20
Stridex Maximum Strength Alcohol Free 20
Stroke Risk Reduction 51
Suave Dandruff Control Shampoo 50
Sucrets Complete Lozenges 46
Sucrets DM Cough Formula Lozenges 46
Sucrets Herbal Lozenges 46
Sucrets ICE 46
Sucrets Sore Throat Lozenges 46
Sudafed 24-Hour Tablets 41
Sudafed Maximum Strength Sinus & Allergy Tablets 41
Sudafed Nasal 12-Hour Tablets 41
Sudafed Nasal 24-Hour Tablets 41
Sudafed Nasal Decongestant Tablets 41
Sudafed OM Sinus Cold Nasal Spray/ OM Sinus Congestion Nasal Spray 59
Sudafed PE Cold & Cough Caplets 41
Sudafed PE Nasal Decongestant Tablets 41
Sudafed PE Nighttime Cold Caplets 41
Sudafed PE Nighttime Nasal Decongestant Tablets 42
Sudafed PE Non-Drying Sinus Caplets 42
Sudafed PE Severe Cold Formula Caplets 41
Sudafed PE Sinus & Allergy Tablets 42
Sudafed PE Sinus Headache Caplets 42
Sudafed PE Tablets 42
Sudafed Sinus Cold 12 Hour Nasal Spray/Sinus Congestion 12 Hour Nasal Spray 59
Sugar-Free Dr Pepper 83
Sugar-Free Mr Pibb 83
SugarTwin 32
Sulisobenzone 84
Summer's Eve Douche 93
Summer's Eve Feminine Cloths 93
Summer's Eve Feminine Wash 93

Sunett 32
Sunscreen 84
Supac Tablets 26
Surfak Liqui-Gels 57
Swab Plus Swabs 69
Sweet'N Low 32
Sweet One 32
Swim Ear Drying Aid 70
Symphytum officinale 106
Systane Liquid Gel Drops 65
Systane Lubricant Eye Drops 65
Systane Nighttime Lubricant Eye
    Ointment 65
Systane Preservative Free Lubricant
    Eye Drops 65
Systane Ultra Lubricant Eye Drops
    65

T

Tab 83
Tagamet HB Tablets 29
Tanacetum parthenium 108
Taraxaci herba 102
Tavist Allergy 12-Hour Relief Tablets
    42
Tea 82
Tearisol Eye Drops 65
Tears Again Eye Drops 65
Tears Again Eye Ointment 65
Tears Again Liquid Gel Drops 65
Tears Naturale Forte Lubricant Eye
    Drops 65
Tears Naturale Free Lubricant Eye
    Drops 65
Tears Naturale II Polyquad Lubricant
    Eye Drops 65
Tears Naturale P.M. Lubricant Eye
    Ointment 65
Tetrasine Eye Drops 65
Tetrazene ES-50 Ultra High-Energy
    Weight Loss Catalyst Capsules 98
Tetrazene KGM-90 Rapid Weight
    Loss Catalyst Capsules 98
Theraflu Cold & Chest Warming
    Relief Liquid 42
Theraflu Cold & Cough Hot Liquid
    42
Theraflu Cold & Sore Throat Hot
    Liquid 42
Theraflu Daytime Severe Cold &
    Cough Caplets 42
Theraflu Daytime Severe Cold &
    Cough Hot Liquid 42
Theraflu Flu & Chest Congestion Hot
    Liquid 42
Theraflu Flu & Sore Throat Hot
    Liquid 42
Theraflu Flu & Sore Throat Relief
    Syrup 42
Theraflu Nighttime Cold & Cough
    Thin Strips 42
Theraflu Nighttime Severe Cold &
    Cough Caplets 42
Theraflu Nighttime Severe Cold &
    Cough Hot Liquid 42
Theraflu Nighttime Warming Relief
    Syrup 42
Theraflu Sugar-Free Nighttime Severe
    Cold & Cough Hot Liquid 42
Theraflu Vapor Patch 46
Thera-Gesic Cream 21
TheraTears Liquid Gel Lubricant Eye
    Gel 65
Thiamin (B1) 95
Thinz Caplets 98
Thinz Tablets 98
Thrive Gum 81
Tiger Balm 21
Tinactin Antifungal Absorbent
    Powder 90
Tinactin Antifungal Cream 90
Tinactin Antifungal Deodorant
    Powder Spray 90
Tinactin Antifungal Jock Itch Powder
    Spray 90
Tinactin Antifungal Liquid Spray 90
Tinactin Antifungal Powder Spray 90
Tinamed Wart Remover 34
Tineacide Antifungal Cream 90
Tinosorb M 84
Tinosorb S 84
Tioconazole 1 Day Vaginal Cream 93
Titanium dioxide 84
Titralac Chewable Tablets 29
Titralac Plus Chewable Tablets 29

T.N. Dickinson's Witch Hazel
Hemorrhoidal Pads 53
Topical Antifungals 89
Topical Wound and Burn Care 91
Topricin Cream 21
Total Acne Control 19
Total Effects Plus Blemish Control
Moisturizer 20
Total Lice Shampoo 71
Transdermis Scar Therapy Topical
Serum 92
Traumeel Ear Drops 70
Traumeel Ointment 21
Traumeel Oral Drops 26
Traumeel Oral Liquid in Vials 26
Traumeel Tablets 26
Treatment Bar 20
Triaminic Chest & Nasal Congestion
Syrup 42
Triaminic Cold & Allergy Liquid 43
Triaminic Cold with Stuffy Nose Thin
Strips 43
Triaminic Cough and Runny Nose
Softchews 43
Triaminic Cough & Sore Throat
Liquid 43
Triaminic Cough & Sore Throat
Softchews 43
Triaminic Day Time Cold & Cough
Liquid 43
Triaminic Decongestant Spray Nasal
& Sinus Congestion 59
Triaminic D Multisymptom Cold
Liquid 43
Triaminic Long-Acting Cough Liquid
43
Triaminic Multisymptom Fever
Liquid 43
Triaminic Nighttime Cold & Cough
Liquid 43
Triaminic Nighttime Cold & Cough
Thin Strips 43
Triaminic Vapor Patch Cough 46
Trifolium pretense 104
Triple Antibiotic Ointment 92
Triptone For Motion Sickness Tablets
61
Trixaicin HP Cream 22
Trolamine salicylate 84

Tronolane Anesthetic Hemorrhoidal
Cream 53
Tronolane Cream 53
Tronolane Suppositories 53
Tucks Anti-Itch Ointment 53
Tucks Hemorrhoidal Ointment 53
Tuck's Medicated Cooling Pads 77
Tucks Medicated Pads 53
Tucks Take Alongs Medicated
Towelettes 53
Tucks Topical Starch Hemorrhoidal
Suppositories 53
Tums Chewable Tablets 30
Tums E-X 750 Chewable Tablets 30
Tums E-X 750 Sugar Free Chewable
Tablets 30
Tums Smoothies Tablets 30
Tums Ultra 1000 Chewable Tablets
30
Twinlab Mega L-Carnitine Tablets 98
Twinlab Metabolift Ephedra Free
Formula Capsules 98
Tylenol 8 Hour Caplets 26
Tylenol Allergy Complete Multi-
Symptom Cool Burst Caplets 43
Tylenol Allergy Complete Nighttime
Cool Burst Caplets 43
Tylenol Allergy Multi-Symptom
Nighttime Cool Burst Caplets 43
Tylenol Allergy Multi-Symptom
Rapid-Release Cool Burst Caplets
43
Tylenol Allergy Multi-Symptom
Rapid-Release Gelcaps 43
Tylenol Arthritis Caplets 26
Tylenol Arthritis Geltabs 26
Tylenol Cold Head Congestion Day-
Night Pack Caplets 43
Tylenol Cold Head Congestion
Daytime Capsules 44
Tylenol Cold Head Congestion
Nighttime Caplets 43
Tylenol Cold Multi-Symptom Day-
Night Pack Caplets 43
Tylenol Cold Multi-Symptom
Daytime Citrus Burst Liquid 44
Tylenol Cold Multi-Symptom
Daytime Rapid-Release Cool Burst
Caplets 44

Tylenol Cold Multi-Symptom Nighttime Cool Burst Caplets 43
Tylenol Cold Multi-Symptom Nighttime Cool Burst Liquid 44
Tylenol Cold Multi-Symptom Rapid-Release Gelcaps 44
Tylenol Cold Multi-Symptom Severe Cool Burst Caplets 44
Tylenol Cold Multi-Symptom Severe Cool Burst Liquid 44
Tylenol Cold Severe Head Congestion Caplets 44
Tylenol Cough & Sore Throat Daytime Liquid 44
Tylenol Cough & Sore Throat Nighttime Cool Burst-Honey Lemon Warming Liquid 44
Tylenol Extra Strength Caplets 26
Tylenol Extra Strength Cool Caplets 26
Tylenol Extra Strength EZ Tablets 26
Tylenol Extra Strength Rapid Blast Liquid 26
Tylenol Extra Strength Rapid-Release Gelcaps 26
Tylenol Regular Strength Tablets 26
Tylenol Severe Allergy Caplets 44
Tylenol Sinus Congestion & Pain Daytime Cool Burst Caplets 44
Tylenol Sinus Congestion & Pain Daytime Gelcaps 44
Tylenol Sinus Congestion & Pain Daytime Rapid-Release Gelcaps 44
Tylenol Sinus Congestion & Pain Nighttime Caplets 43
Tylenol Sinus Congestion & Pain Nighttime Gelcaps 44
Tylenol Sinus Congestion & Severe Pain Cool Burst Caplets 44
Tylenol Sinus Severe Congestion Daytime Cool Burst Caplets 44

U

Ultra Brite Toothpaste 69
Ultra Daily Face Wash 19
Ultra Deep Pore Cleansing Pads 19
Ultra Diet Pep Tablets 98
Ultraprin Tablets 26

Ultra Tears 65
Uristat Tablets 26
Urtica dioica and Urtica urens 104
Uvae ursi folium 112
Uvasorb HEB 84
Uva Ursi Leaf 112
Uvinul A Plus 84
Uvinul T 150 85

V

Vaccinium macrocarpon 107
Vaccinium myrtillus 105
Vaginal Products 93
Vagisil Anti-Itch Cream/Medicated Wipes 93
Vagisil Foaming Wash 93
Vagisil Intimate Moisturizer 93
Vagistat 1 Vaginal Cream 93
Vagistat 3 Combination Pack 94
Vagistat 3 Vaginal Cream 94
Valerian 114
Valerianae radix 112
Valerian Root 112
Vanquish Caplets 26
Vaseline 92
Vaseline Intensive Care Aloe Cool & Fresh Moisturizing Lotion 77
Vaseline Intensive Care Cocoa Butter Deep Conditioning Lotion 77
Vaseline Intensive Care Healthy Hand & Nail Lotion 77
Vaseline Intensive Care Lotion Total Moisture 77
Vaseline Intensive Rescue Clinical Therapy Lotion 77, 88
Vaseline Intensive Rescue Healing Hand Cream 77
Vaseline Intensive Rescue Heal & Repair Balm 77
Vaseline Intensive Rescue Moisture Locking Butter 77
Vaseline Intensive Rescue Moisture Locking Lotion 77
Vaseline Jelly 77
VasoClear-A Eye Drops 65
VasoClear Eye Drops 65
Vasocon A Eye Drops 65
Verbena officinalis 104

Vervain 104, 113
Vicks Cough Drops 46
Vicks DayQuil Cold & Flu Relief
    Liquicaps 44
Vicks DayQuil Cold & Flu Relief
    Liquid 44
Vicks DayQuil Cough Liquid 44
Vicks DayQuil Sinus Liquicaps 44
Vicks Formula 44 Custom Care
    Chesty Cough Liquid 44
Vicks Formula 44 Custom Care
    Congestion Liquid 45
Vicks Formula 44 Custom Care
    Cough & Cold PM Liquid 45
Vicks Formula 44 Custom Care Dry
    Cough Suppressant Liquid 45
Vicks Formula 44 Custom Care Sore
    Throat Lozenges 46
Vicks NyQuil Cold & Flu Relief
    Liquid 45
Vicks NyQuil Cold & Relief
    Liquicaps 45
Vicks NyQuil Cough Liquid 45
Vicks NyQuil D Liquid 45
Vicks Nyquil Sinus Liquicaps 45
Vicks Sinex 12 Hour Nasal Spray/12
    Hour Ultra Fine Mist for Sinus
    Relief 59
Vicks Sinex Nasal Spray For Sinus
    Relief 59
Vicks VapoInhaler 46
Vicks VapoRub Cream 47
Vicks VapoRub Ointment 47
Vicks VapoSteam 47
Visine A.C. Astringent Redness
    Reliever Drops 65
Visine-A Eye Drops 65
Visine Allergy Relief Drops 66
Visine L.R. Redness Reliever Drops
    66
Visine Maximum Redness Relief 66
Visine Moisturizing Drops 66
Visine Multi-Symptom Relief 66
Visine Original Drops 66
Visine Pure Tears Lubricant Eye
    Drops 66
Visine Tired Eye Relief 66
Visine Total Eye Soothing Wipes 66
Vitamin A 95

Vitamin B6 95
Vitamin B12 95
Vitamin C 95
Vitamin D 95
Vitamin E 95
Vitamin K 95
Vitamins 95
Vitamins A & D Ointment 77
Vitex 102
Vitis vinifera 109
Viva-Drops 66
Vivarin Tablets 82
Vomiting 61

W

Wake-Up Call Tablets 23
Wart 34
Wartner Freezing Wart Remover 34
Wart-Off Liquid 34
Weight Management 5, 96
Wild Child Quit Nits Cream 71
Wild Child Quit Nits Spray 71
Witch Hazel 78
Wound Wash Sterile Saline Spray 92
Wyanoids-HC Rectal Suppositories
    53

X

Xtreme Lean Advanced Formula
    Ephedra Free Capsules 98

Y

Yeast Gard Douche 94
Yeast Gard Feminine Wash 94
Yeast Gard Gel Treatment 94
Yeast Gard Suppositories 94

Z

Zaditor Eye Drops 66
Zantac 75 Tablets 30
Zantac 150 Tablets 30
Zantrex 3 Ephedrine Free Tablets 98
ZAPZYT Acne Wash Treatment For
    Face & Body 20

ZAPZYT Maximum Strength Acne
Treatment Gel 20
Zeasorb Super Absorbent Antifungal
Powder 90
Zegerid OTC Tablets 30
Zicam Allergy Relief Homeopathic
Nasal Solution Pump 59
Zicam Allergy Relief Nasal Gel 59
Zicam Allergy Relief with Cooling
Menthol Gel Swabs 60
Zicam Extreme Congestion Relief
Liquid Nasal Spray 60
Zicam Intense Sinus Relief Liquid
Nasal Spray 60
Zicam No-Drip Liquid Nasal Gel 60
Zicam Sinus Relief Liquid Nasal Gel
60
Zilactin-B 6 Hour Canker & Mouth
Sore Relief Gel 69
Zilactin-B Canker Sore Gel 69
Zilactin-B Long Lasting Mouth Sore
Gel 69
Zilactin Early Relief Cold Sore Gel
69
Zilactin -L Cold Sore Early Relief
Liquid 69
Zilactin Lip Balm 69
Zilactin Tooth and Gum Instant Pain
Reliever 69
Zinc 95
Zincfrin Eye Drops 66
Zincon Medicated Dandruff
Shampoo 50
Zinc oxide 85
Zinc Oxide Ointment 78, 88
Zingiber officinale 108
ZNP Shampoo Bar 50
Zostrix Arthritis Cream 22
Zyrtec-D Tablets 45
Zyrtec Itchy Eye Drops 66
Zyrtec Tablets 45

Author Biography

Frank J. Nice, RPh, DPA, CPHP

Dr. Frank J. Nice has practiced as a consultant, lecturer, and author on medications and breastfeeding for 40 years. He holds a Bachelor's Degree in Pharmacy, a Masters Degree in Pharmacy Administration, and Masters and Doctorate Degrees in Public Administration. Dr. Nice holds Certification in Public Health Pharmacy and is registered as a pharmacist in Pennsylvania, Maine, Arizona, and Maryland. He practiced at the NIH for 30 years and currently serves as a pharmacist and project manager at the FDA.

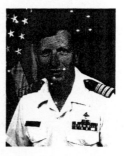

Dr. Nice has organized and participated in over two dozen medical missions to the country of Haiti. He retired from the US Public Health Service after 30 years of service as a Commissioned Officer and pharmacist. He served 20 years of that time at the National Institutes of Health's Clinical Neurosciences Program as Assistant Program Director.

Dr. Nice has published over two dozen peer-reviewed articles on the use of prescription medications, Over-the-Counter (OTC) products, and herbals during breastfeeding, in addition to articles and book chapters on the use of power, epilepsy, and work characteristics of healthcare professionals. He continues to provide consultations, lectures, and presentations to the breastfeeding community and to serve the poor of Haiti.